With thanks to our
good friend at
Peoples Bank ~

Esther E. Hansen

90 YEARS YOUNG!

Adventures in Wellness

ESTHER E. HANSEN

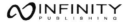

All rights reserved. No part of this book shall be reproduced or transmitted in any form or by any means, electronic, mechanical, magnetic, photographic including photocopying, recording or by any information storage and retrieval system, without prior written permission of the publisher. No patent liability is assumed with respect to the use of the information contained herein. Although every precaution has been taken in the preparation of this book, the publisher and author assume no responsibility for errors or omissions. Neither is any liability assumed for damages resulting from the use of the information contained herein.

Copyright © 2012 by Esther E. Hansen

ISBN 978-0-7414-7585-5 Paperback
ISBN 978-0-7414-7586-2 eBook

Cover Design by Joseph Daily with Maria Cadorette

Printed in the United States of America

Published June 2012

INFINITY PUBLISHING
1094 New DeHaven Street, Suite 100
West Conshohocken, PA 19428-2713
Toll-free (877) BUY BOOK
Local Phone (610) 941-9999
Fax (610) 941-9959
Info@buybooksontheweb.com
www.buybooksontheweb.com

TABLE OF CONTENTS

Introduction

Chapter 1: "You Are What you Eat!" 1

Chapter 2: "Go Out and Play" 10

Chapter 3: "Here's what Mom would have done." 19

Chapter 4: "You are deprived of every vitamin known to man." ... 28

Chapter 5: Health Advice from the Twelfth Century 37

Chapter 6: Meeting a Healer in Our Time 46

Chapter 7: The First Modern Physician! 54

Chapter 8: A Revolutionary Discovery 64

Chapter 9: Health Help from the Past in New Hands 72

Chapter 10: Healing at Our Fingertips 81

Chapter 11: The Touch of Healing 91

Chapter 12: Natural Healing Science Pioneers 100

Chapter 13: What Did You Say? 108

Chapter 14: What is The Healing Code? 117

Chapter 15: Chiropractic and Acupuncture 126

Chapter 16: The Miracle of Water 134

Chapter 17: Health Hazards in the World Around Us....................144

Chapter 18: Staying Healthy Through the Years 154

Chapter 19: Tomorrow's Physician...164

Chapter 20: Health of Body, Mind and Spirit 172

Bibliography..181

INTRODUCTION

Yes, I'm a senior! I never thought I'd reach the age of 90! Well, surprise! In only a few years that could happen! So many years spent on this planet!

Thanks to my dear friend Janet in Holland I am now able to share in print some of what I have learned about being well. I am deeply grateful to her and to other friends who have extended generous interest and support through their written contributions to the book.

I'm thankful for everything I've experienced in all these years. I'm thankful for being physically and mentally in good health. That and more! I want to share some of the things I've learned. I want to introduce some of the people I've met, in print or in real life. I want to tell you what they taught me about wellness. It has all been good and useful.

One thing I've learned is so elementary that I may risk offending the reader by mentioning it. It's a commonly-shared experience upon recovering from some major or minor physical upset to realize how much better we function when we feel good. We think more clearly. Everyday pleasures mean more to us. We are much more ready to participate in life as we know it. Wellness is important! It's important to learn how to be as well as possible.

No two of us walk the exact same road. What I have found on my road might help you to find something on yours that is right for you. I wish you pleasure in seeking, patience with the detours on which I may lead you, and joy in finding and experiencing wellness!

Esther E. Hansen

CHAPTER ONE

"You Are What you Eat!"

"You are what you eat!" It was my Danish mother's favorite English saying, and we heard it every day, for sure, during the years when my sister and I were growing up in the 30's and early 40's. She may have heard it on the radio--there was a man called Victor Lindlahr who used the term in his radio talks. Possibly she had picked it up in early writings by Adelle Davis, whose works first appeared in England and may well have been made available in Danish translation. However it reached my mother's English vocabulary, she made it her own.

Eating was important in our family, and our mother made certain that eating was a pleasure. Not only was eating itself a good thing, she saw to it that whatever you ate that came from her kitchen was good for you!

There was an inherent respect for food in the family, which came, in part, from our Danish tradition. The word that invites people to come to a meal—"Vaersgo" in abbreviated form (actually "be so good") is untranslatable, but it implies that something good is about to happen. It means that those who hear about it are welcome. And the Danish words, familiar from earliest childhood on, that come at the end of the meal are "thank you for the food," --- "Tak for mad!" Any of our friends who shared a meal with us soon learned those words and knew what they meant.

We gave thanks for food and respected it. There was no such thing as "junk food". Junk was something you threw away when it was worn out or otherwise not wanted. The word would never have been applied to food. I remember, actually, feeling a dreadful sense of guilt and shame because my mother had fixed too much lunch for me, and I quietly threw away a piece of bread and whatever was on it. You didn't ever throw away food!

There might be special treats from one of the wagons that came through the neighborhood—an ice cream truck with a cheerful bell that heralded its coming, and the glorious fragrance that informed us that the popcorn wagon was on its way down our street. With luck you might be given a nickel for a treat; at school that entailed an agonized choice: Would it be a large pickle or an Eskimo pie---a square of vanilla ice cream covered with chocolate? Either one of these cost a nickel. (I belong to the generation that is still shocked by today's two-dollar ice cream cone.)

Of course there were home-made cookies, especially at Christmas time when a new fragrance greeted us each day on coming home from school: pepper nuts and brown cookies, vanilla wreaths, "Finnish bread", currant cakes and others. Christmas Eve brought the beloved familiar scents of roast duck with apples and prunes, and red cabbage, cooked with vinegar and currant jelly. It was often prepared a day in advance of the feast, like the Christmas cake, which was baked ahead of time to be enjoyed on Christmas morning.

A special treat that our friends loved too was "aeggesnaps" --- egg in a cup or a glass stirred and stirred with sugar and cocoa and eaten with delight by a roomful of happy kids, each with her own self-made treat. It was soft, smooth and delicious. An old friend still mentions "eggysnaps" with that same delight still in her voice.

And there were the freebies that we never told grown ups about—I can still feel the crunch of winter's icicles against my teeth, and the summertime sweetness of honeysuckle on my tongue. Such were the treasures found by those of us who made our way home from school via back alleys.

There were others who gathered as family groups around their tables. The lady next door had a brood of boys, and the "Yoo Hoo" with which she summoned them home for dinner was heard for at least a mile round about us. In that house too eating was a shared experience, and there were jobs associated with it: shelling peas, husking corn, setting the table. Food was one of the things that made you feel secure--- loved and protected.

And let's not forget: it also kept you healthy! My mother believed in good nutrition, and her example became clear in my memory and my sister's. It encouraged us to do likewise on our own; it was passed on to the generation that followed. Vegetables and fruit, meat and fish, fruit and other sugar-free desserts were carefully chosen and prepared. Variety was welcomed and expected; meals were well planned and food was always appetizing and eye pleasing.

A traveling salesman sold my mother a set of wonderful pots and pans. They were made of stainless steel - no danger of aluminum invading the meals that came from her kitchen! She was able to prepare vegetables with only a little water, and what water was left over went into the soup pot to add extra vitamins and minerals. Nothing was ever over-cooked. Meat and fish that was braised or fried came out super delicious from that frying pan. Mom was happy to brag about her "Silver Seal pots and pans".

Of course we remember special meals from those good times at home. There were "frikadeller" the traditional Danish meat balls made of a mixture of ground meats, flour, eggs and milk—beaten and beaten until all was thoroughly and smoothly mixed. The meat patties could be sautéed on the pan, and were served with potatoes and vegetables. The leftovers would be stored away in the ice box to reappear in neat slices for the open - faced sandwiches we always had for lunch. Like other foods, the open - faced sandwiches were always decorated—with pickles, with parsley, with slices of tomato. Pleasure for the eye was important too.

The force meat could also appear in the stuffed cabbage, served with melted butter, that was a special family favorite. Or it was turned into small meat balls and served in curry sauce, with lots of onions. Another favorite in our family was a beautiful platter of cooked vegetables (I see it in memory-- a bright palette of colors, green beans and golden carrots, white potatoes and yellow corn.)

The veggies were served with butter of a different sort, softened until it could be stirred, and called, of course, "stirred butter"

Green peas were often served with cubes of carrots, generously mixed with parsley. Sometimes we added cubes of ham and called the dish "Ruskumsnusk." Whether that was a dish known to other Danes or a family specialty, I am not sure.

Roast lamb was the Easter specialty. It was seasoned with parsley and served with cucumber salad. Roast chicken was often a Sunday treat, which of course always turned into chicken soup with cardamom-flavored dumplings. We had fish from local waters – shad roe from the Potomac was especially good, and fish balls that came to us in cans from Norway. We liked calf's liver with onions; beef tongue was delicious.

Fruits were common as desserts: strawberries and blueberries, blackberries and raspberries in season, slices of cantaloupe served with grapes and a sprinkle of sugar. Summer fruits were crushed, thickened with corn starch and served with sugar and cream. It was called "Rodgrod" (red porridge) or as our good friends liked to term it in their attempt at Danish, "Ooey Gooey with Flooey." Whatever it was called it was GOOD. Spoonfuls of fruit preserves went into the buttermilk soup, flavored with sugar and lemon, that was often a favored summer dessert.

Fruits also appeared, both summer and winter, in fruit soups of various kinds made of fresh, canned or dried fruits and usually thickened with a bit of tapioca. Apple cake was served with lots of whipped cream and recognized by our friends as what they called "Brown Betty."

Thanks to my mother's willingness to add to her Danish recipe repertoire, we also had pies. As a newlywed in this country, my mother had carefully observed through her kitchen window the black lady next door making pies. She soon tried it out and found that it was easy to replicate what the lady did. Lemon meringue pie was my father's favorite, and my mom became expert at making it.

She also learned to imitate American birthday cakes, so that we could each order whatever had become our favorite. The Danish version, usually chosen by grownups, was a delicate white cake with a layer of macaroons and fruit jelly along with lots of whipped cream. Sometimes there was a birthday "Kringle"-- a giant size pretzel-shaped coffee cake, sprinkled with sugar and almonds.

Guests often joined us at the table, and this was especially true at Christmas. Christmas dinner was unchangingly ever the same and wonderful. Danes knew exactly what to expect, and Americans were agreeably surprised. Christmas dinner always came on Christmas Eve. There was love and joyful recognition of the holiness of that evening among us at the table. If any failed to perceive it, they had, at the very least, a most satisfactory meal.

It began with risengrod, translated as rice porridge, which was simply rice cooked with milk for hours and hours. Started on the stove, the porridge, when it began to thicken, was transferred in its pot to a down comfort, where it spent the afternoon all snug and warm and slowly cooking. Just before dinner was served the porridge returned to the kitchen, where it was heated again and milk added if necessary.

As we were seated, my mother poured the porridge into a silver serving dish. She held up a blanched almond and explained that she was now placing this almond in the porridge. Whoever found it in his bowl would be given a special prize. Each one of us was to serve himself. No fair stirring around and peeking for the almond! A pat of butter was placed in the center of each serving; it was sprinkled with sugar and cinnamon and topped with fruit sauce.

There was happy suspense at the table until someone declared, "Here it is! I've got it!" In our family the almond finder was awarded a pig—a pig made of almond paste, for my mother was good at modeling. In later years, in our own homes, we had searched out clay, glass or porcelain pigs to use for this award.

Roast duck, stuffed with apples and prunes followed the rice porridge. There was red cabbage in its special Christmas version that everyone loved. There were glazed potatoes and cranberry sauce,

There was plenty of brown gravy and plenty of seconds for those who wanted them.

Coffee was served for adults at the end of the meal, and heaps of cookies and home made candies, especially marzipan fruits and vegetables. The meal was unforgettable and delicious Always the same, every year again!

* * * * *

Did our mother know about vitamins and other supplements? Definitely! Like many others who grew up in these years we were given cod liver oil. And I'll always remember the vitamin pill we were given in addition: we always had to rush for school, and sometimes were almost late because my poor sister had such trouble swallowing that vitamin pill.

Vitamins and other supplements were important. Food had to be cooked right in order to keep its values intact. Food had to be nutritious, but it also had to be delicious. It had to look good and taste good. Those were my mother's basic beliefs, the ones we knew and respected and learned to live by. They were the ones we ultimately made our own.

We wonder where Mom got her knowledge. Was it part of her Danish upbringing and culture? Possibly. There is no easy way to know that any more. Her generation has passed on. and ours is going. When her writing and activity became known, my mother joined the many who were followers of Adelle Davis, a name still known and respected by some.

Who was this lady? She studied in California and earned advanced degrees in biochemistry from USC and Columbia. After the Second World War this wonderful American woman became widely known for her writing, her lectures, her enthusiastic activity. She worked as a consulting nutritionist with doctors in California.

During her lifetime she stated that she had planned individual diets for over 20,000 patients suffering from almost every known disease. With her help, patients with incurable diseases were helped to recover or improve significantly. Through her research and knowledge simple health measures, still well known, have influenced our diet and our health habits today. All those shelves of yogurt at the grocery, for instance, are probably there thanks to Adelle Davis.

Her name became a household word through her books, *Let's Eat Right to Keep Fit, Let's Get Well, Let's Have Healthy Children, Let's Cook it Right*, and others. Her writings first appeared in England. *Optimum Health*, which came out in 1935, is the one I've wondered about---did my mother somehow get hold of that book? The date coincides with my childhood years and could have influenced the healthful diet I experienced as a child.

Be that as it may, what's important is to have a look at the basic premises brought forth and disseminated by this great lady, Adelle Davis---.the ones that played a part in my life.

Adelle Davis was a biochemist. She plowed her way through endless research studies focused on the effects of vitamins and minerals, on animals and human beings She learned about the dramatic effects of vitamin deficiencies and the extraordinary healing powers of large amounts of vitamins that might be needed by a human being.

Working in consultation with doctors, she was able to plan for specific needs of patients suffering from all kinds of human ills Multiple experiences with the abnormal increased her understanding of normal needs. She was able to give sound advice about vitamins and minerals to help us fulfill our normal daily needs.

Food was not simply something to fill our stomachs when we were hungry. What was important was the nutrition in that food, which was what we needed to keep us feeling well and healthy. The right nutrients could make us well if we were sick. But we can also get sick because of not getting the vitamins and minerals needed to keep us well. Not all diseases are caused by bacteria.

But food should also be delicious. It should be a pleasure to consume the substances we need to sustain the health of our bodies.

And people could learn to cook food properly in order to ensure preservation of the all-important food values. Vegetables could be steamed with very small amounts of water, or dropped into shallow boiling water so none of its goodness would be lost. Even the cooking water could be kept and used---it has food value too. Adelle Davis liked to describe good food as "having all the known nutrients."

We needed to cut down our sugar consumption. Sweets, we were told, take away our appetite for the good food our bodies need.

Adelle Davis advised pregnant women not to "eat for two", as they might have been told. She told them to eat normally and then increase their intake of vitamins and minerals in the third trimester of pregnancy.

She gave attention to weight loss and told those trying to lose weight, "the more you eat the more you want to eat; the less you eat, the less you care to eat."

Adelle Davis is a name still recognized and remembered happily by some of us. She raised concerns about food safety and health that some people objected to at the time. But her views have long since been vindicated. They are among the issues being dealt with seriously by science and health practitioners today. In the kitchen good mothers have long since recognized the common sense of what Adelle Davis taught and practiced.

In scores of kitchens across the continent –across the world actually-- women paid attention and families experienced better health because of Adelle Davis My mother was one whose cooking habits were affected. The good Danish food we ate was prepared with careful attention to its food values. My sister and I grew up healthy.

My father chuckled at his wife's preoccupation with vitamins and minerals. But he never protested, for the food we ate was the best. It was delicious, and if it was also good for you, well, so much the better. "Tak for mad," said he. "Tak, min skat!" (Thank you, my treasure!)

90 Years Young!

* * * * *

For me it has been good to follow in my mother's footsteps with regard to food. Many others have likewise learned from their own mothers what was later practiced in their own homes. Many authors, since Adelle Davis was so active, have emphasized, as she did, that the kind of food we put in our physical bodies gives us the physical strength, the energy and stamina and the well being we need to be what we want to be as human beings.

Good food is important and good food makes good people.

CHAPTER TWO

"Go Out and Play"

"Go out and play!" was what the young were told when I was a child.

<u>Out</u> was where you went to play. <u>Out</u> was where you played tag and jumped rope. It was where you drew hopscotch games on the sidewalk, and circles for playing jacks. You found pebbles there for playing stone school and good spots for hide and seek.

If you had a park across the street, you had a great place for egg rolling at Easter and sledding when the same hills were covered with snow. In spring you found violets in the woods there, and heaped up leaves in the autumn for jumping into and rolling around. <u>Out</u> was where you took your roller skates and scooters and wagons for all kinds of active play.

<u>Out</u> was where you played "doctor" with your dolls in the play house, and gave plays that you made up and presented for whoever wanted to come. If you had a father like ours with "good ideas," you might go out for ice skating because one very cold winter he managed to create a skating rink in the back yard.

Unless it was freezing cold or pouring rain, "out" was a great place to be. Other kids were out there too, which was usually a benefit. I venture to say that our generation was in better health because of all the good time we spent outdoors.

Walking was something the whole family believed in; it was my father's cure-all exercise. At 94 he was still making use of this lifetime favorite. I expect to be making use of it myself at that age.

90 Years Young!

The rest of us never thought about the health benefits of walking; it was pleasant, it was easy to do, and it was fun if the whole family did it together. Actually, researchers agree on its benefits. They tell us that those who walk regularly live longer and are more free of disease than folks who are sedentary. They are less likely to catch cold. Studies even indicate that walking reduces the risk of developing cancer and glaucoma. Even walking on a treadmill is beneficial -- it seems to relieve depression. We didn't have treadmills or pedometers, but never mind, walking was good and it was good for us.

Dog walkers have always been out there, of course. But today lots of other folks seem to have joined up with the dog walkers. Some just step outside the door in comfortable shoes and walk for ten minutes. In our town we have sidewalks, which helps. "Nothing like a good sidewalk," my father used to say.

Others go at it more systematically, and that's good too. They establish a regular routine and take their ten minute walk every day 4 or 5 days, or a week. Then they increase the time by 5 minutes and speed up the tempo on the last 5 minutes. They establish a pattern: 10 minutes of regular walking, then smaller, faster steps for 5 minutes. Gradually they increase the time, building up to two daily walks of 20 some minutes each—about 45 minutes a day. Impressive!

* * * * *

I was no great fan of organized sport; I was quick to find ways of avoiding having to come up to bat when we played baseball at school. (Teacher looks the other way – you go to the end of the line.)

It was no better when I got to college. As a freshman I endured hockey-- no way to escape the thundering herd in that sport ! Dodge and volley ball were better, and I survived them. Later, the only thing that would fit into my schedule was tennis. Alas, I was not cut out for that either! After endless dismal rounds, the teacher, who really was a peach -- I liked her -- looked at me with a hopeless sigh. "Hansen, how many years have you been <u>taking</u> tennis?" "Almost three, Miss Kriener." She sighed again. "I don't believe it," she said, shaking her head.

Badminton was better; it was more like dancing and that was good. But it was a rare treat, reserved for special times, whatever they were. Dancing—yes! Near the end of my college career something called "modern dance" appeared on my schedule. It was glorious! It called for individual movement. It sent you flying across the room in beautiful, uninhibited movement. Your body was twisting and turning, bending and swaying in leaps and bounds. It was not dependent upon what anyone else did. I loved it! And for the first time ever, I earned an "A" in "physical education."

* * * * *

And then there was Mascha! She brought us a whole new and different kind of physical education. It involved the whole body. It made us realize that we were much more than bones and joints and muscles. It made us aware of our bodies and what they were, what they could do, how much they played a part in every move and action that we carried out all day long. She was a teacher like no other teacher we ever had or would have.

Mascha was a survivor of the holocaust. She had lost everyone and everything that was dear to her. The one sister that was left lived with her husband and their daughter in New York City. Mascha came there, and ultimately she came to Washington, where I lived with my parents. She made the terrible years she had survived come alive for us. It was really true; the ghastly things we had read about were real. They had deeply affected this human soul, this special person who came to mean so very much to us.

The new kind of physical education she shared with us was born out of the experiences that had made up her life in Europe. In Germany, where her Russian-born parents had settled, she had been educated in Dalcroze eurhythmics, with their emphasis on free and natural movements and creative expression. She had studied with Mary Wigman, who had such a great influence on dancing, whose work contributed so much to what I was to know in college as "modern dance." In Poland, where she stayed briefly on her flight from Germany, she studied ballet.

In Denmark, to which she escaped and spent some years, she was befriended by Gerda Alexander, whose body education was to gain worldwide attention. In homes, schools, factories, offices everywhere she taught people to use their bodies in the right way to carry out normal human tasks. Office and factory workers were given time during the work day for exercise classes that taught them how to make better use of their bodies to serve the needs of the companies they worked for. There were no more aching backs, stiff joints and sore wrists and fingers. Cramps and tension were gone. Musicians in the Copenhagen symphony orchestra felt better and played better thanks to their work with Gerda Alexander.

Swedish massage was added to Mascha's repertoire; she learned it in Sweden, to which she fled in the last days of the Second World War. When I met her in Denmark she had returned there and was planning the last step in her journey to the United States. I was able to help her get established and set up her practice in Washington when she finally settled there.

Mascha had learned in multiple ways about the human body. She was a competent teacher and a wise and loving human being. We who became her pupils were fortunate to have her.

She taught us body awareness; we learned to identify and connect with our body parts and to use them to become strong and flexible. We learned how to relax, not only when we were still, but to relax in the right way when we were carrying out normal movements. We learned how to identify the source of discomfort if we didn't feel well. In her classes we experienced a sense of well being in every part of our bodies.

I felt a sense of grace and strength and power in my own body and loved having the opportunity to help my teacher in working with children. A little Brazilian boy was one of her pupils. He had asthma, was underweight and frail looking. His mother, who had been in one of Mascha's classes, wondered if he might benefit from working with her. I joined the two in what to him was just fun and play. Some months later, when the family returned to Brazil, Celso showed me with his fingers how thin he used to be. "I used to be such a skinny little thing," he said, "but now I am a strong boy." And he showed me his arm muscle proudly.

A ten-year-old girl who was one of my reading pupils suffered from the anxiety and tension of the over-scheduled modern child. (She loved Sundays because there was nothing scheduled on that day.) Learning how to relax with passive exercises and active movements was to her too just "fun and games." She too understood how this kind of help was useful to her. "I'll need you till I'm married," she said once. She didn't though; her reading also improved significantly.

*****

Both Mascha and I were interested in yoga, and we traveled to France to participate in a course given by a man who was among those from India who were bringing the practice of yoga to the western world. We respected the work of Selva Rajan Yesudian. The yogic practice of sensing and feeling the changes going on in the body, both externally and internally, felt familiar. We observed the skin as it began to tingle and become warm. We felt the stretching of muscles as we maintained the fixed positions. We felt the release of tension as the body relaxed into a posture. "My will power and my resistance are developing from moment to moment" chanted the man. And we felt and believed it.

Yoga is carried out primarily through static postures. In Denmark we experienced the quite different approach of Moshe Feldenkrais in his "awareness through movement." In a class we experienced a portion of the wellness he had learned to give to patients seriously disabled by physical disease and injury.

Through my friend Mascha I experienced and was given exposure to many systematic expressions of body training. I was surprised and delighted by them. I experienced in my body the difference between active and passive in so many ways: tension and relaxation, perceiving all the possibilities in the body, and giving them expression in my own individual ways. Leaping uninhibited across a room and lying on the floor realizing that I had a spine, arms and legs that could sense and experience, that could stretch and bend and move at my command. Lungs that could consciously take in oxygen related to the energy that suffused my body and was channeled to every part of the me that is physical.

I began to understand that physical part of myself, and how it is related to all the sensory organs—to see and hear with appreciation and understanding, to feel with full awareness, to express my own being in response to all that I saw and heard, and sensed in so many different ways!

I have thought about what they had in common—everything from what we now call "modern dance", or did when I was in college, to yoga, to training of the body through the instruction of Gerda Alexander and Moshe Feldenkrais.

What was it that they had in common? Surely it was first of all respect for the human body and responsibility for its well being. What I learned from Mascha and from the various systems to which I was exposed was body awareness.

Like all of us in the western world I watched the Olympic performers, and, like many others, I was fascinated by the ice skaters-- in particular the ice dancers. Without professional knowledge, I recognized the best of them. They gave absolute pleasure by the bodily harmony they exhibited, which seemed to be an integral part of their being. We watched dancers and knew which ones were the best because they demonstrated the best that a human being can show—absolute harmony of the outer, physical being and the inner being that we most often keep to ourselves. The young woman who performed immediately after the passing of her beloved mother expressed that so movingly. The emotions she showed in her performance with so much grace and beauty were felt by all who watched her.

In the same way, I watch the people who pass my windows each day on the new sidewalk that has recently been constructed in my village. There they go: old ones and young ones, mothers and children, young people hand in hand, older folk with canes, proud dads with baby buggies, dog owners walking their canine pals. There are not many who captivate me with the grace of their physical movement. (Actually, I have been most interested of late in watching a lady who is physically handicapped, walking with controlled determination to master the limitations imposed by her limbs.)

Usually the dogs are happy and uninhibited when they go by. I think of my Happy, the beagle I had, who lived up so completely to her name. She was in charge of our walk, no doubt of that, and sometimes she made onlookers chuckle when she sat down resolutely to protest my decision about the way we should walk. But once we set off again (on her chosen way) she was all joy from nose to wagging tail.

Part of our joy when we visit the zoo is in our observation, conscious or not, of the absolute beauty of animal movement. They are in harmony with nature. We often are not.

What Mascha taught us, as do the various systems that train and cultivate physical well-being, was and is the knowledge and expression of that harmony. We probably had it as kids when we were sent outside to play. As grownups we have to learn it all over again.

* * * * *

In Washington, when I lived there, I saw Martha Graham in what must have been one of the last performances of her life. I wonder what I was able to tell people about that extraordinary dancer. Did I manage to express the total wonder I felt when I saw her? In memory I still see her dancing. And I know that age does not have to stand in the way of bodily grace and beauty.

As I entered the "golden years," I slacked off a bit on organized exercise. Of course, like other dog owners, I went for the twice-daily walks with my canine buddy. Walking is good exercise, but I had long since learned that a healthy body requires more than that.

In a magazine discovered in my niece's home in Arizona there was an article about "The Five Tibetans." The small group of exercises so designated was described and pictured. Hmm-could I do these? They seemed to offer important benefits for a minimal expenditure of time and effort.

The first was simply standing up straight, arms spread, and spinning around clockwise. That one was easy for me. I managed 10 rotations without difficulty.

The second, lying on the back with arms alongside the body and lifting both legs up to a ninety degree angle resembled exercises I had experienced before. It too was not a challenge for me.

Likewise, the third, in kneeling position, which involved arching the body, including the head, backward. However I wasn't sure I'd want to do it 21 times, as suggested.

The last two exercises were challenging: the fourth one required lifting the body from a sitting position into a bridge balanced on hands and feet, and the fifth elevated the body from a face down into an elevated triangle supported by hands and feet as a base.

Of course I wanted to try them out at once and ultimately to read more about them. What I learned then and later was that the exercises had been brought to the attention of the western world through a little book called *The Five Rites of Rejuvenation* by Peter Kelder, written in 1939. According to his engaging account, the "rites" had been discovered somewhere in the depths of Tibet by a retired British army officer. This gentleman was said to have returned "rejuvenated" from Tibet after learning and performing the exercises taught him by lamas in a monastery there.

Whether the story told by Peter Kelder was fact or fiction was perhaps never verified. However, it caught the attention of many who wanted to stem the aging process and improve the health and strength of body and mind. Obviously of yogic origin, the "five

Tibetans", as they became known, were based on sound principles. And they were effective.

Each of them was to be performed 21 times. I tried that but didn't care to do it regularly. I settled for 7 (except for spinning, which I did 12 times). Mastering the last two exercises required patience and persistence, but once they were acquired it was easy to add them to my repertoire. When mastered, the series is quick and easy to do. I've conducted my modified version almost without fail every morning I have no doubt this contributes to my feeling of wellness.

Proponents of the system are everywhere. In Europe I heard of an elderly lady so determined to make use of the exercises that she was using a small stool and a chair for support as she mastered them. Here at home, when I told my chiropractor about them he said, with startled delight, "You do the Tibetans?"

In old age I no longer dance, but I can control my body. It is a pleasure to move my body and its parts. I was startled and surprised when somebody said to me, "The first thing I thought when I met you was how nicely you moved-- like a dancer." Me? -— A dancer?

A dancer I am not, but I have experienced the joy of dancing. I have been exposed to competitive sport, yoga and many special kinds of exercise. Each one taught me something I needed for my life in a physical body here on this earth.

That body must serve my needs. It must serve my needs however limited they may be by age or impediment. I want to move with dignity. I want to recognize the signals in my body if something needs special attention. I want to take pleasure in the physical body that I have in whatever way is right for me. We can all experience that satisfaction!

CHAPTER THREE

"Here's what Mom would have done."

All over the world sensible moms have known what to do to keep their families in good health. They were right there, on their own, or supplementing the work of the recognized healers. What they knew and did contributed in good measure to what has come to be known as folk medicine. We knew about it in the days when I was a child. We knew that Mom could be depended on to make us feel better, to know at once what was the right thing to do when one of us was not up to par. The doctor was our friend when we needed him. Our mother, like good mothers everywhere, was his invaluable helper.

Of course the mothers knew. They had learned from their mothers, and those grandmothers had learned from their mothers. Sensible measures had been passed down through the generations. Bumps and scrapes, stings and bites, burns and every other kind of childhood ill were all attended to. Much later we would say to someone in a new generation, "I know just what to do. Here's what my mother would have done."

Many wise, simple practices have helped us to survive and thrive in spite of all the expected and unexpected threats to our well-being. The things we knew about were not well-kept secrets. They were familiar remedies that most everyone knew about.

Someone with a cold would find himself tucked into bed with cozy, warm blankets, waiting for a "hot toddy" made with steaming tea and spiked with honey. (Grown up people could expect a little brandy in theirs.) Then there was chicken soup, the benefits of which have now been proven by those who need to prove why things really work. None of us cared to know why chicken soup worked for colds; we just knew that it did. It was good, and it made us feel good. Our chests had been rubbed with Vicks Vaporub and our throats were wrapped in woolen scarves. If you coughed you were given horehound drops. None of us knew them to contain a natural product, a bitter mint with downy leaves. We didn't know why they worked; we just knew that they did.

Some maladies were associated with holidays: too much cookie sampling along with the excitement that preceded Christmas Eve in our house could lead to upset stomachs, for which the standard remedy was oatmeal cooked very soft, with applesauce added. What a soothing remedy that was! I remember passing that information on to the mother of a child I was teaching. He came to me on the day after Halloween, looking….well, did you ever see a <u>green</u> child?

If we had trouble sleeping we knew that a cup of warm milk with honey dissolved in it would send us off to dreamland; a toothache could be controlled with cloves from the spice container in the pantry. One of those long spiky leaves of aloe vera could be sliced open and applied to burns, wounds and insect bites to speed the healing.

Bits and pieces of information about the healing powers of plants, trees, roots and flowers found their way into my childhood days. I remember hearing from my mother that chamomile could be helpful for menstrual cramps. My grandmother had said that chamomile was so beneficial for women that every woman who found a chamomile plant should curtsy deeply. For me, beyond the time of curtsies, the wonderful knowledge of healing help from the world of nature was reserved for the future. I will tell about those discoveries in another chapter.

* * * * *

I think one of the valuable skills that I learned from my mother was to keep my eyes open for simple remedies in the world around me. Pharmaceuticals were not necessary to preserve my good health or solve a health problem if I had one. I was excited to learn about Vitamin C for instance, and how effective it was in combating the common cold. I found that it worked for me, regardless of what the nay-sayers might declare. For me it proved to be useful to know after I had begun life on my own and returned occasionally to visit my parents. I did not want to bring home any kind of "bug" to my father, who suffered from asthma and emphysema. A number of times I experienced, if awakened in the night by a significant sniffle or a rough feeling in the throat that a few thousand units of vitamin C could chase away the symptoms.

* * * * *

I ran across an old-fashioned home remedy that I was glad to pass on to friends who shared a problem I had. I had moved to Ohio, where I found that during the growing season my eyes were bothered by allergies to some of the growing things. For a couple of years I just lived with it and hoped for some nice home remedy that wouldn't cost an arm and a leg.

The ophthalmologist had offered me a prescription for a pharmaceutical product. I said "no thanks" to the offer and later was delighted to discover this old home remedy that actually works. The best part of it is that the ingredients are probably right there on your kitchen shelf and are super easy to combine. (Like me, you may have experienced the helpful home remedy that sends you off to the health food store, with reference book in hand, to search for the ingredients.}

Here is the easy recipe for this good remedy:

> You will need: 5 parts water, 2 parts honey, 1 part apple cider vinegar. Shake it all up together and put it in a small jar to be used with an eye dropper.

If you have one of those nice little brown bottles that come with a dropper, that's perfect. The brown bottle protects the mixture so that it doesn't spoil. My nice little plain glass jar was collecting mold, so I had to throw away part of my remedy. Then I found a brown bottle with a built-in dropper. (It had contained stevia extract.) It's much handier that way and I have no more trouble with spoiling. (Don't make more than enough for about two weeks at a time.)

A drop or two when I need it has solved my eye allergy problem. The eye doctor approves; there's no harm done to the eye. And I can enjoy the beautiful days of spring-summer-fall with clear eyes and a happy heart.

* * * * *

Friends shared their favorite health tips with me. Exchanging such tips can be a useful and interesting project. Sharing my eye allergy treatment brought to mind a friend's family remedy for sties and other simple eye problems. A dripping tea bag was squeezed dry, cooled and applied to the eye as a soothing poultice.

Another friend shared her tips about hot and cold compresses: a boiled egg can be used for a small hot compress, a bag of frozen peas or other veggies serves well for a cold one.

I learned from a friend and proved it to be true that myrrh is good for any problems, like canker sores, in the mouth. I keep myrrh gum capsules available and open them to slide the powdery substance onto my hand and apply it on a finger to a canker sore in the mouth; It is soon cured.

An office worker has a standard remedy for paper cuts. She cleans up the cut, dries it off and sprinkles on some powdered clove. It acts as a painkiller and apparently also prevents infection Keep some in the office alongside your scotch tape, pens and pencils!

Some tips came by e-mail. Here are a few:

"Hi, this is how I help myself" read the greeting. The tips followed.

- "COLDS, FLU AND SORE THROAT: Gargle with lightly salted warm water. At that first sign of tingling in the nose I sniff the saltwater up into my nose. Repeat two or three times. Or use a Neti pot. It works great for flushing out the sinuses with saltwater. (Ask in the health food store about a Neti pot. You can get one there.)

- "ARTHRITIS PAIN: Mix one Tablespoon of liquid fruit pectin into half a cup of grape juice, wine, or herb tea, once a day. This works on one kind of arthritis pain. If it doesn't work, ask in the health food store about cell salts and get #4.

- "ITCHY EARS: Vinegar (white or brown. I always keep a squirt bottle in the bathroom. Just squirt it in. Instant relief! The doctor gave me a vinegar and alcohol mixture over 40 years ago when my ears were driving me nuts. It worked instantly. When I ran out I mixed it myself and finally just used vinegar. It works!!!

- "JOINT DISCOMFORT, and URINARY URGENCY: Dried cranberries or cranberry juice. A glucosamine-chondroitin product like Elations from WalMart or the health food store can also be good.

- "STOMACH DISCOMFORT: After eating, or later on, suspecting food poisoning or intestinal flu, I take 1 iablespoon of "Swedish Bitters" diluted with warm water in a juice glass. Repeat as needed. (Ask at the health food store for Swedish Bitters.) It is important to do this as soon as you notice something isn't right. If you're on coumadin, ask your doctor. (My husband would take Jaeger Meister (from the liquor store)—1 shot glass. It tastes better and works too!)

- "BRUISING and PAIN: Swedish Bitter packs work wonders!!! I have used this amazing liquid for over 25 years. It has never let me down. I have also used it for gum and ear inflammation.

"Since I've been introduced to Essential Oils, MELROSE OIL has become my #1 First Aid remedy. I use it for all minor wounds, inflammation on the gums, insect bites, rashes and sores, cuts, fungus, and tissue regeneration. It can also be used on dogs and horses.

"To build and regulate the immune system, the main thing I have found is TRANSFER FACTOR. It is highly praised among many, including cancer patients. It is powerful yet safe. My motto is "first do no harm" and I believe Transfer Factor fits that description. It has helped me in a big way with my leukemia!!!"

* * * * *

The specific products mentioned by my friend in her e-mail will be discussed at greater length here and in some of the chapters that follow. Swedish Bitters, Transfer Factor and essential oils are products that we might well wish our parents had known and used as we do today. They can become faithful friends, providing dependable answers to many everyday health problems.

The wonderful product called Swedish Bitters is mentioned among my friend's favorite remedies. Many of us have learned to look for it at health food stores. It did actually originate in Sweden centuries ago. It was the result of the research and work of a Swedish doctor, Dr. Samst, who proved the effectiveness of his product by living to a great old age. Apparently he persuaded his family to use the wonder cure as well, for they too all lived to be very old.

The Swedish doctor didn't get the credit for his work though. It was Paracelsus, a renowned physician who lived in the 16th century, who stumbled upon the work of Dr Samst and let anyone who would listen know about it. Eventually it reached the hands of an Austrian woman in our time, Maria Treben. Thanks to the Swedish doctor and to Paracelsus, not to mention the kind help of a neighbor who helped to cure her of typhoid fever, Maria Treben learned about Swedish Bitters and told the world about it in practice and in print.

Maria Treben's work is worth knowing about. I'll discuss it again in one of the forthcoming chapters.

* * * * *

90 Years Young!

The daily paper we find at our doorstep sometimes provides the very answer someone is looking for in the column featuring health tips from Dr. Gott, a medical columnist who is a practicing physiclan.

One column offered the following:

"Soap Remedy Helps Ex-Marine

"DEAR Dr. GOTT: As a mud Marine in World War II, I had my gluteus maximus blown away, femur broken, etc. I was told I would be in a wheelchair by the time I was 40 years old after being in a body cast for nine months. I'm close to 84. I do 100 pushups, swim, weight lift, etc., but my left hip is painful. I have no joint. It all calcified from immobilization for nine months in the hospital. But the good news is, by sleeping with a bar of soap on the gluteus maximus muscle, 90 percent of the pain I experienced upon awakening in the morning has left. No clinical reason. But I play golf, walk with a cane, and lead a normal, active life. I fly a plane and am able to use the left rudder despite a 3-inch shortening of my left leg. My reason for writing is, please tell people the soap treatment does help arthritis sufferers. A friend has arthritis in his left hand. I told him of the 'soap' treatment. He put a cake of soap in a glove and wore it in bed. It has helped him a great amount –- no cure, but a real help.

"DEAR READER: Thank you for suggesting yet another use for the soap treatment. ·Your story is intriguing. You may achieve better results from rubbing castor oil into the affected area. Many arthritis sufferers swear by this treatment, which is safe, easy and inexpensive."

DR GOTT's best known remedies were summarized in one newspaper column:

- "SOAP FOR NOCTURNAL LEG GRAMPS: Simply pace a bar of soap, unwrapped, under the bottom sheet of your bed near your legs. This remedy takes effect immediately.

- CASTOR OIL FOR ARTHRITIS: Rub a small amount of castor oil into the affected joint or joints, morning and night. May take effect immediately, or full results may not be seen for up to four days.

- GRAPE JUICE AND CERTO FOR ARTHRITIS: Place 1 to 2 tablespoons of liquid Certo (or any brand pectin) in 8 ounces of purple grape juice. Drink up to three times a day. May take up to four days for full results.

- VICKS VAPORUB: For nail fungus, simply clip the nail as far back as possible without causing pain, and rub Vicks onto the nail and surrounding skin twice a day. This may take months before results are visible. For fungal infections of the skin (athlete's foot, jock itch, etc.) or psoriasis, simply rub a small amount of Vicks onto the affected area twice a day. May take up to a week to clear.

- CHERRIES FOR GOUT: Eat six to 10 cherries daily as a preventive or 10 to 15 at the start of and during the gout attack. Reduces the length and pain of the attack.

- COLON COCKTAIL FOR CONSTIPATION: Equal portions of apple sauce, bran and prune juice. Take 1 to 2 tablespoons each morning. May take up to 19 days to be fully effective.

- BREWER'S YEAST FOR MOSQUITOES. Take one 7.5 milligram tablet each day to repel mosquitoes. Usually works immediately.

- EAR PAIN: Sweet oil and garlic oil work wonders for ear pain caused by infection. Simply warm and place a few drops into the ear. Results should be immediate"

* * * * *

There must be heaps of home remedies for hiccups. Our favorite aunt in Denmark had a cure that always worked. She took the child gently by the hand and directed her gaze upon him. The hiccuper held his breath expectantly—and the hiccups were gone. Whether this worked anywhere else for anyone but her I wouldn't know.

A remedy that has found its way into medical textbooks is a spoonful of just regular sugar, without water or any other liquid to wash it down.

Another old remedy is this one: You put a knife or a long-handled spoon into a glass of water. You drink the water while holding the utensil next to your temple. I haven't tried it, but they say it works.

* * * * *

The extraordinary American psychic, Edgar Cayce, provided specific individual advice to those who became his patients. Included in his recommendations are some simple procedures that have proved to be helpful to others. Among these is his head and neck exercise. It is a simple routine that anyone can easily learn and remember for daily use. It is to be performed carefully and slowly.

You sit erect. Bend the head forward three times.
        Then bend the head back three times.
        Then to the right side three times.
        Then to the left side three times.
        Then circle the head each way three times.

This not only makes your head and neck feel good. Performed on a regular basis it is said to reduce stress, improve circulation, and detoxify the system.

* * * * *

CHAPTER FOUR

"You are deprived of every vitamin known to man."

Like other young people, I took for granted my good health, and soon forgot all the good things that had brought it about. It was not until I was on my own, away from all the nice nourishing food, the supplements that kept me well and staved off disease, that I had the opportunity to arrive at independent and personal conclusions about health and how to maintain it.

For the first few months after I left my parents, I lived alone in a rented room. It was pleasant enough, and I was glad to have peace and quiet there to work on the master's thesis I was turning out. I fixed my breakfast in the kitchen and carried it on a tray up the stairs to my little haven under the eaves. Other meals I took at school--the same hot meal that was prepared and served for the children every day at lunch time--and in the evening I often ate at a local family-style restaurant where foods were kept on a steam table so they were hot and ready to serve.

I was eating well enough I thought. Vitamins? Whoever bothered to think of those!

I was contented, but not very well physically. I experienced extreme fatigue that sometimes kept me away from my teaching job or sent me home early before the end of the school day. Doctors, I thought, were for "old people" like my parents or for those who were really sick. But after a while it seemed that a doctor might be needed.

The good man was not able to identify my problem, but he suggested antibiotics and kept proposing new ones when the first of them failed to put me back on my feet.

My good friend Dorothy, who was interested in the thesis, and concerned about my health, invited me to stay with her. She and her husband lived in a comfortable old house only a few blocks from where I was staying. It was good to be there; they were kind, interesting people I was fond of them and never felt myself to be an imposition.

"Why do you have that rash?" Dorothy wanted to know. I had no idea. She advised that I see a doctor she knew--a dermatologist. On my return from there I announced: "I have an atopic dermatitis." "Well, I could have told you that!" said Dorothy, who was an ophthalmologist.

In her home I was given a good diet, the same sort of foods I had been accustomed to at home. I had a little more energy and managed to hold out through whole school days. If Dorothy ever thought of vitamins she never brought up the subject. She was not bossy, and would have considered it my own business.

Then we met the Greek doctor. She was at a lecture we attended to which I had been invited along with Dorothy. The two of them chatted afterwards and arranged to meet again for dinner. I was asked to join them.

The doctor from Greece was definitely a personality. She had a robust figure and a kind face. As we talked, she told about her early experiences in this country. She had come to find out more about the learning disabled children, in whom she was keenly interested. Apparently there were many of them here in the states, and she wanted to explore why this was the case.

At first she wondered about birthing. Did something go wrong at the birth of these disabled learners? She was permitted to be present at births all over this country. Her pronouncement: "It was beau- ti - ful!" There was obviously nothing wrong with the way we brought children into the world in this country.

Then her research focused on experiments with guinea pigs. She exposed them to smoke from cigarettes. She gave them alcohol.

Guess what! The guinea pigs were adversely affected. They became "learning disabled." They failed to perform as guinea pigs should.

"What is wrong with these human children?" asked the Greek doctor. "What is the cause of their learning problems?" She was quick to respond to her own question. The answer was self evident: to her: "The drinking of the father, the smoking of the mother!"

To us she said, "Just raise guinea pigs and expose them to alcohol and tobacco smoke. You'll soon see what happens!" And she added an aside of her own: "Many of these children are conceived at holiday times. But not at Thanksgiving; then people go home to Mama."

* * * * *

When she heard that this same doctor had established a practice in our city, Dorothy urged me to go and see her. There were the usual tests, including blood, urine, and hair testing. Some samples were sent off for assessment of vitamin content in the body. What in the world would that show?

Like those I had already heard from her, her words when I came back for the second appointment, were clear and straightforward: "You are deficient in every vitamin known to man!"

Me? Me who thought I had grown up healthy, whose mother fed me cod liver oil and vitamin supplements. Who ate nutritious, carefully prepared food served by a loving, conscientious mother. Me who knew all about eating properly. Me, deficient in vitamins?

Enlightenment came along free of charge with the vitamin shots, given to compensate for my deficiencies, and massive multivitamin supplements that followed. I had to admit that I was not eating entirely the way I used to at home. I had forgotten all about vitamins or any other supplements. And the food prepared in school and restaurant kitchens was kept warm on steam tables, certain to extract any nutritious value from the good veggies and other foods there.

Needless to say, I became a healthier person. Dorothy safeguarded the food value in the meals I had in her home. I was back on health-conscious eating and vitamin supplements.

* * * * *

Here I was then, a real-life demonstration of life with and without multivitamins. I learned to use the term, and to understand that it comprised the familiar lettered vitamins plus minerals and other substances essential for the health of the human body.

Slowly but surely I began to pay attention to what made a person healthy. I had always taken health for granted. Obviously my mom was right. There was no doubt that my new friend the Greek doctor had knowledge that was valid and important. Vitamin supplements had made me strong and healthy again.

I began to wonder what other experts had to say. I did some reading and eventually discovered the wonderful world of the internet. I began to explore its endless corridors of information and misinformation. There were claims and counterclaims, wise words and foolish ones.

"Use your head," they used to tell me. It was time to do so in a new way. I learned which voices to trust and which could not be trusted. I sorted out fact and fiction. There were independent studies that were trustworthy; they were interesting, and they made sense to me. I looked for scientific research.

In 2009 a large group of women in our country--over 500--between the ages of 35 and 74 was divided into two groups. One group was given multi-vitamins; the other was not. Each group was tested before and after a prolonged period. The vitamin takers showed clearly measurable indications that they would live longer and be healthier than those who did not receive supplements.

In China there had been a much larger study, conducted over a much longer period of time. More than 29,000 city residents were involved. The focus was on a specific type of cancer common in that area of the country. Those who took part in the study were given multivitamins for six years. During the years that followed they were tested regularly to assess the ongoing results of the supplements they had received. The vitamin-takers were significantly more healthy than others in the same city who did not receive any supplements. Even ten years later the tests still indicated a reduced risk of chronic disease and early death. And the Chinese people who took the multivitamins also showed a reduced risk of cancer.

Scientific research confirmed what I had learned from experience. Multivitamins make you feel better, avoid disease, and live longer!

My own experience fed the desire to know more. With my explorations the familiar vitamins I had so long taken for granted gained new importance. For Instance, the "sunshine vitamin," Vitamin D, was an old friend long touted by the dairy world as especially necessary and desirable. I learned that it is indeed critically important for helping us avoid colds and flu, not to mention heart attack, rheumatoid arthritis and depression.

And it has been discovered that the vast majority of Americans are seriously deficient in this precious vitamin. It was reassuring to know that as a dog owner who has always believed in walking my pet regularly I was naturally exposed to lots of sunshine—the best way to absorb lots of Vitamin D. Cyclists and joggers along with gardeners also soak it up in their favorite activities, but those who spend most of their lives indoors obviously need to boost their sunshine vitamin levels in the supplements they take.

And newcomers took a bow on the stage of my awareness. There was CoQ10--a vitamin-like substance that has been studied, used and recommended for many conditions. And Omega 3 oils, which are really fatty acids that may help lower the risk of some diseases, including heart disease.

In reliable multivitamins there are many components that were new to me, backed by years of scrupulous scientific research. Making a wise choice of a dependable health company from which to purchase multivitamins became a new responsibility.

Early in our present century scientific research verified what, by then was already becoming common knowledge. Scientists were urging health professionals to advise patients, old and young, to eat a healthy diet and to be sure to get their vitamins!

Even the prestigious Journal of the American Medical Association declared that all adults should take vitamin supplements to help them be well and prevent chronic diseases. Quite a different tune from what was heard in the past!

* * * * *

My mom always used to long for a nice pill that would contain all the food value a person should have, without all the work involved in cooking! Dinner in a pill! She thought it a wonderful idea. Recalling the wonderful meals I enjoyed at her table in my childhood and youth, I had to disagree!

Well, we haven't come to that point, but with vitamins it's a different story. Multivitamins do come in neat pills or capsules, and they sort of bridge the gap between what we do eat and what we should eat.

Actually, it's a fact that most of us don't get all the vitamins and other supplements we need in our food. Even if we consume the minimum recommendation of five servings of fruit and vegetables every day, it's actually harder than it used to be to make sure we're getting the full benefits from them that we did in the past.

Science has discovered that we'd have to eat a much larger amount of fruits and vegetables to receive the same food value that we got in a much smaller amount when we were kids. When this information was divulged even the scientists were amazed. They had demonstrated a decline in all the major nutrients in produce over the last 50 years. It ranged all the way from 6 percent, for protein, to 20 percent for vitamin C and as much as 38 percent for some of the other nutrients. That makes multivitamins doubly important And multivitamins, though they may not always measure up to what we have a right to expect in terms of quality, are available in every drug store.

Choosing the right multivitamin, I discovered, entails some responsibility on our part. Clever marketers know how to promote their products. They know how to advertise so that a customer is quick to make a purchase. Those products most prominently advertised are not necessarily the best. I was shocked to learn that some brands, when tested, were revealed to simply pass through the human digestive system without being absorbed in the blood stream. They were never dissolved but were excreted intact, providing no benefit whatsoever.

Obviously, the right multivitamins are good for us. Those whose quality can't be trusted will do us no good at all.

* * * * *

All over the world, university labs and government programs confirm the importance of the food we grow. Produce protects against heart disease and cancer; it helps to reduce the risk of stroke, high blood pressure, birth defects and diabetes. The high fiber in fruits and vegetables helps to prevent obesity. Apparently we haven't even begun to search out and recognize all the benefits found in the growing things that should be a regular portion of our daily diet.

But, as already mentioned, there is a dark side to this cheerful news. In order to derive the same benefits that our parents and grandparents got from their fruit and vegetables in average portions, we would have to consume huge quantities of the same natural products.

Farmers have obligingly worked to supply the increasing demand for their wares by growing large sized fruits and vegetables faster than ever. In order to do so they have used chemical fertilizers and insecticides. And that has reduced the benefits of vitamins, minerals, calcium and other components in the foods we grow.

Not only the growing things, but the soil itself is less healthy than it was in the past. Humus, the essential foundation of living soil, built up over centuries by the decomposition of plants and leaves, is no longer as it was in the past. It has been weakened by artificial fertilizers and polluted by chemicals that have brought on fungal diseases and insect attacks previously unknown.

To me it was a shock to learn that there is pure, beautiful soil in the basin of the Amazon that is today just as it was 2000 years ago! In our country, actually everywhere in the world, there is no such soil. It has been weakened and deprived so that it no longer serves as the basis for health-giving produce as it used to do centuries ago.

Modern agriculture tries to supply the deficit by adding chemicals to the soil. Some of these chemical fertilizers kill off the various soil bacteria and beneficial fungus and earthworms, all of which support the humus that is so important to insure healthy growth.

This background helps to explain the growing popularity of organic foods in our grocery stores and the increasing attention given to supplying the needs we have come to recognize with nutritional supplements in daily pill dosages.

* * * * *

What about organic foods? A friend told me recently about going into a new grocery store and finding a "gorgeous display" of organic produce. Apparently the company found it well worth their while to cater to the wishes of those who seek out those fruits and vegetables.

This development, which would seem to be an increasing trend, will also lower the expense associated with organically grown produce.

Meanwhile, is it really worth the extra expense? If you can afford it, the answer is yes. Organic produce has not been exposed to chemical insecticides or fertilizers. The plants have produced their own defenses to protect themselves and this increases their food value for human beings. The food value that we expect to find in growing things has been preserved intact. It comes to us just the way food would come from our own gardens if we were in a position to grow it there.

Not all of us can afford it though. Should we give up fruits and vegetables because we can't afford the best? Of course not. We can shop carefully, look for good color in our produce, choose smaller rather than larger items, make sure to eat things when they're fresh. That means only a week old, or less, so that more of the food value is preserved. We can avoid greens and other vegetables that come all nicely sliced or shredded—they're less nutritious.

We can be sure to wash fruits and vegetables carefully, perhaps with a little vinegar in the water. We can peel them to get rid of whatever they may have been sprayed with, and then cook them giving attention to simple, basic rules. Most vegetables are best steamed. Roasting is a good idea too. It makes some things like tomatoes or broccoli release more of their nutrients.

Frozen produce has almost as much food value as fresh, unless it has been treated with additives to preserve the fresh taste. Except for tomatoes you won't find much food value in canned food.

Eating well is no longer the simple matter it used to be. A person who wants to experience strength and physical well-being has to be well-informed and attentive to his personal needs. It requires thoughtful individual effort. Emotional growth cannot be disregarded. Many have learned that simple foods enjoyed in a loving atmosphere can far surpass elegant fare served at banquet tables.

If we are willing to make the effort, we can all eat a healthy, balanced diet, no matter our age or the physical challenges we may have to live with. We can all enjoy good food. We can enjoy life!

For the sake of clarity, this chapter has omitted certain health hazards found in modern food. These will be discussed in the chapter titled "Health Hazards in the World Around Us."

CHAPTER FIVE

Health Advice from the Twelfth Century

Experience had made me curious about health and physical well- being. I wondered about the past, the years of knowledge and folk wisdom, passed down from one generation to the next. In checking out the past I had not expected to go back so far.

But here I was, over 900 years back in time, to a woman whose name is not totally unknown to me. Surely the name has a familiar ring. ...Yes, I noticed it on a CD. She was known for her music. Her beautiful devotional music is still played and enjoyed today. Now I learned to my utter surprise that her knowledge of medicine is the basis of a new branch of modern medical practice in Germany.

Who was she? What did she know, and how did we find out about it?

She was born long ago in Germany, near the town of Bingen in the year 1098. She is venerated as a saint in the Roman Catholic Church: Hildegard of Bingen. What does she have to do with medicine?

Hildegard was the tenth child born to parents of the nobility who lived on a country estate in a pleasant area of rolling hills and farmland. The little girl "saw things" from her earliest childhood on- -not only the loveliness of nature in trees, fields and flowers. This child saw more than that, and as a little one she shared what she saw with anyone who wanted to listen. She saw pictures of distant places and times and described them accurately in detail. She could tell about things that were totally unknown to others. Once, for instance, she foretold correctly the color of a calf as yet unborn.

The child became her parents' "gift to God." They were Christians who decided to give this tenth child as a tithe to the church. When she was 8 years old the little girl was taken to live with a devout woman, Jutta, who was a recluse. Her dwelling place, where she lived like a nun, was attached to the nearby monastery, which was directed and run by men. Sister Jutta became the child's friend and mentor. She taught her young pupil to read and write, and to sing psalms of praise. Music and needlework were also included in her instruction.

When she was 14 Hildegard became, along with Jutta, an anchorite of the monastery. Ultimately Jutta became the prioress of a separate Benedictine cloister for women in which she and Hildegard were nuns. When Jutta died 12 years later, it was Hildegard who assumed this leading role of the 20 women who had joined the cloister.

Even when she was a child, other women had come to live in the vicinity of Hildegard, who had so many extraordinary things to tell. To the nuns who became members of the cloister her visions gradually played an active and important part in their lives.

The young woman's health was fragile; she lapsed sometimes into periods of unconsciousness from which she awoke with new stories to tell of the wonderful things she had seen and experienced. The gifted prioress became known for her visions.

They had never been kept a secret. She shared them with her confessor, who advised her to write down her experiences and show them to the abbot who had authority over the cloister. The abbot showed what she wrote to the local archbishop, who joined in urging her to continue writing. During the next ten years Hildegard penned a report of 25 visions. These are said to sum up the Christian doctrine of the history of salvation.

As time went on the nature of her visions was greatly intensified. She was 43 when she began to see a "heavenly screen" of light in front of her by day and night. She described it as a "shimmering cloud of light." From it issued messages of many kinds that were meaningful. She no longer spoke so freely of those things that were revealed to her. A heavenly voice told her to write down all that she saw and heard. This she did, and at the same time she was writing hymns.

Eventually a songbook of 77 chants, hymns, and other musical works appeared among her writings. These were played and sung in her own time and have been rediscovered in our day. They have been played and recorded for thousands of people to hear and enjoy all over the world.

Thus began Hildegard's remarkable writings. When the voice of Pope Eugenius was added to the many who urged her to set down in writing everything that was revealed to her, it dispelled her misgivings about putting her knowledge into print. She set down detailed theological works discussing the gospels and Christianity, some of them in the literary form of poetry or plays. She told of the creation of angels, of the sun, moon and stars *God is the source of all life*, she wrote.

She wrote of human beings, their virtues and vices, and of the cosmos as the home for humanity. All things were in order at the beginning of creation. And human beings lived in support of creation and in harmony with it, so there was no sickness or evil. These were brought about by man himself.

She was sensitively aware of nature, and its four elements, fire and air, earth and water. *All things in nature are associated with the four elements*, she wrote, *and so, inevitably, are we human beings, and so is healing and the healing arts.*

Although her health was sometimes compromised, while her visions often separated her from the physical world around her, she was constantly related in a positive way to its needs, and ever determined in action to support, enrich and improve them.

Realizing the necessity of herself maintaining active leadership and direction of the nuns who had attached themselves to her, she achieved permission to establish a new convent under her rule. There in Rutisberg, not far from her native Bingen, she instructed them in the Benedictine rule of life. Her life, and that of the nuns associated with her, was far less comfortable physically, than it had been in the first convent, but all of them were totally dedicated to serve God and the needs of their fellow human beings. Under Hildegard's rule they were more free to act as they saw fit.

By then her writings had become widely known. Papal verification of her prophecies had been given and thousands of pilgrims sought her out in person. Others corresponded with her. Among her writings 300 letters have been found. To people in every station of life--kings and queens, prominent clergy, including the pope--she gladly offered advice and counsel.

Always willing to share the knowledge that had been given her, she also traveled extensively to one place after another. Well into her 70's this remarkable woman was sought out to appear in person at places far distant from her own convent. She willingly journeyed far and wide by boat, on horseback or on foot in all weathers and seasons to share her knowledge and wisdom with others. It is not hard to imagine the physical stress of such journeys, long before our modern age of convenient, luxury transportation.

Until her death at 81, Hildegard continued to supervise the convent at Bingen, which had grown to include about 50 nuns. New quarters were required as a basis for the activity of 30 additional nuns. This work was also supervised by Hildegard.

To this day her music compositions are played. She was made a saint by the Roman Catholic church and is known and venerated. Yet her medical knowledge has remained ignored, unknown and unused, until very recently with the research and enlightened activity in Germany of physicians there. "Hildegard medicine" has become a familiar term in that country. Much of the work of Hildegard physicians has been translated into English. Translators are at work to insure that others may benefit from that knowledge all over the world.

Only in very recent decades has her valuable knowledge become known through the work of a German doctor, Dr Gottfried Hertzka, who has worked clinically with Hildegard's theories for thirty years. Dr. Wighard Strehlow, a research chemist who now works with Dr. Hertzka, translated his work into English. In Germany many doctors now know and practice "Hildegard Medicine."

Why were her copious writings about medicine ignored? Was it assumed, perhaps, that the dear lady could have little to share in this field?—that whatever she had to say would hardly go beyond what any woman might have learned from her mother or other women mentors? Had she picked up folk wisdom in the gardens of the convent, heard others discuss the merits of herbs, roots, stems and flowers? Had she herself benefited, when she was ill, from remedies known by those who tended her? All this might easily have been thought or believed by those who found value in her other writings.

While all these elements might have contributed to her store of knowledge, Hildegard herself was quite specific about the source of her medical wisdom. Centuries before her, Hippocrates, the "father of physicians," had declared that his knowledge came from "divine ancestors.'. Hildegard wrote quite plainly that life comes from God. *Life from God comes to us in plants, animals and precious stones.* Her knowledge about life, about health and healing, *"came from God."*

Those who began to explore the saint's writings and seek out the source of her wisdom found these words clearly stated by Hildegard. They gave new weight and meaning to the words extracted centuries later from Hildegard's writings by a practicing physician and those who have worked with him in Germany.

She offered nearly 2000 remedies and health suggestions. They included not only herbal remedies, but prescriptions and detailed instruction regarding bloodletting, saunas and baths as well as specific kinds of massage. Human emotions were emphasized both in diagnosis and treatment. Nutrition was deemed important for maintaining and restoring health. Her descriptions were clear and rational and, when tested in our time by doctors who followed them conscientiously, they were proven to work.

In two areas the words she transmitted might have been written today. The first is in respect to cancer. The origin and appearance of cancer are exactly described as has been proven by modern science. The pre-cancerous state that is present in advance of the development of cancer is clearly delineated. The effect of stress on its development is emphasized, as has been carefully explored and studied in our time by another German physician. Patients are advised to build up bodily resistance so that cancer will be less likely to develop.

Does all this sound familiar? It does if one has read any modern writings about cancer.

The second very important area in Hildegard's writings about medicine concerns detoxification. The importance of maintaining health through avoiding nutritional poisons or ridding the body of poisons so that it may be healed is emphasized. These substances--strawberries, pork and coffee--are considered by her to be nutritional poisons Modern man would be quick to add many others: air and noise pollution, food additives, excessive stress among them.

Another area in Hildegard's writings that is widely recognized in today's world is the importance of our immune system. We know that the immune system protects us from external poisons like bacteria, viruses, toxins and allergens. It also defends us from pathogens in the body itself that can make us sick. Our strongest weapon against these formidable enemies is our own immune system. Hildegard called it the "militia dei"--God's military.

Through the work in Germany of Dr. Hertzka, who has made extensive use of "Hildegard medicine" and who, along with others in his country, is conducting multiple successful treatments with it, this ancient wisdom is extensively known in our time. It is now available also in English, through the skillful work of an able translator. Hldegard's writings reveal understanding of the basic causes of health and sickness.

Hildegard believed that everything you eat and drink either strengthens or harms your health and well- being. The basic diet she recommended to maintain health contained meat and much seafood, fresh vegetables, whole grains and fruits, especially those in season. Spelt was strongly favored, and was described by Hildegard as the very best grain, producing not only "firm flesh and good blood," but "a happy mind and a good spirit."

Moderation in all things was stressed; one drink was deemed good during a meal. Beer and wine were acceptable, in moderation. A plain diet, she said, can be delicious and healthful. Eating right is more important than medicine.

* * * * *

In the extraordinary new world of health care that is coming into being in this century, this woman's voice from the 12rh century is heard again. It speaks with unquestioned authority. It speaks out of unlimited depths of knowledge and conviction. Hildegard of Bingen was not interested in scientific research. She said, "I have never dedicated myself to the human studies of the learned."

The learned of today have a high level of scientific knowledge. Quantum physics has opened an unlimited array of doors to new understandings and significant developments in the world of health.

And now, just at this time, there are those who give ear to that voice from the past and the woman who had such a remarkable understanding of health and sickness. She said "Everywhere in creation there are mysterious healing forces, which no person can know unless they have been revealed by God.'

Hildegard's knowledge, she declared, came from God. Life from God, she said, is transmitted into the plants, animals, precious stones that are used in healing. She knew that treatment of those who are sick required the removal of the roots of the problem, not the treatment of its symptoms.

Those healers who have heard her voice and responded with eager interest by practicing "Hildegard Medicine" no doubt explore, catalog and utilize the specific healing arts recorded in her writing. I and others like me, who do not count ourselves among the "learned," can yet fully understand the basic principles on which her work, and the new healing art that bears her name, are based.

Hildegard believed very strongly that we are personally responsible for our own health. Learn to trust your physician, she said, acknowledge when their help is needed, but learn to be your own physician in many ways. Gradually we can learn to do it.

Learn to give up the things that are recognized as harmful to your health and physical vitality. In our century there are many daily poisons that can sap our strength. Tobacco is one. Others are excess coffee, spirits, addictive drugs or junk food. Each might present a daily challenge for someone to overcome.

I recall with a personal sense of joy that my father gave up smoking when he was 65. His doctor had suggested that if he really wanted to live to a reasonably healthy old age it would be necessary to abandon his beloved pipe. He didn't think it over very long; he decided to live without it, and went on to live a "reasonably healthy" old age--94. He continued to enjoy his daily walks, and I was glad to have him all those extra years!

Learn to eat well and enjoy good food. The food you choose to eat can contribute much to your health. Hildegard did not speak of vitamins, but she knew the value of a correct and balanced diet. She would have agreed with what Adelle Davis declared centuries later: "You are what you eat."

Learn to take more enjoyment in your five senses. See and hear all that the natural world has to offer you. Exercise your body in whatever way is right for you, be it simply in walking, or in dancing, swimming, riding and other active sports. Use your talents in art and crafts of many kinds. Connect with the world of nature by caring for animals or gardening, be it only in a pot of flowers on the window sill.

I remember the gifted writer from the Philippines, who gave similar advice to a college class. I have forgotten his name, but not his words. He spoke of his native home, which was close to beautiful mountains. Often he said to his children, "Have you seen the mountains today?" All of us have some kind of "mountains" near at hand. I remember that when I lived in the big city I rejoiced in the art museums and concerts--available without charge there.

Learn to balance activity with rest, especially restful, beneficial sleep. It can play a very important part in our physical and emotional well- being.

Above all we must believe in God, "the essence of all good, creator and lord of the natural order of things." said Hildegard. Then, as she states, we can be "old and filled with life" and can take the great step into the everlasting state in "full freedom and beauty."

CHAPTER SIX

Meeting a Healer in Our Time

Already I have introduced so many who played an important part in my wellness adventures. Early on there was a knowledgeable woman from California, whose wisdom about how and what to eat became important to me. There was a Greek doctor who underscored the value of vitamins and other supplements for the human body. There was the good lady who applied that knowledge in daily life to retrieve my wellness. There was a refugee from Hitler's oppression who taught me how to know and value the body itself. Back in the 12th century there was one who became recognized as a saint long before her knowledge of healing gained widespread recognition.

Always in the background of my life experiences well into early adulthood was a cousin who was born and lived in Denmark, my parents' native land. As a toddler I recognized her at once. She was my cousin, the daughter of my mother's sister. She was 15 when I was 2. We looked at each other and each of us thought, "What a wonderful person!"

When, as a child, I visited with my mother in Denmark, Rigmor was always there. On our last visit before the Second World War she was living and teaching at a school whose exotic setting was the Castle of Jaegerspris. The castle was the central building of a home and school for orphaned children, There my cousin lived in a small apartment, From its window she could look out on the peaceful Danish countryside, secure from the stresses and demands that became part of life in the Nazi occupation beginning in April, 1940.

I was thrilled to visit the beloved cousin who now lived in a castle. It was exciting to see the "fire escapes" in each of the rooms--large wicker baskets equipped with stout ropes to provide rescue from a burning building. Best of all its attractions was the secret room accessible from my cousin's apartment. There was an iron hatch through which one could jump down into the classroom below--a detail that would later prove very useful to another castle resident who came to take refuge in the castle.

That resident, whom I would later come to know as Sister Rosa, was to play an important role in one of my many "adventures in wellness."

It is important to tell her story here, not only because her life touched upon mine. It is important because it shows how the threads of disaster, in the right hands, can be used to serve a good purpose.

The woman who became "an illegal guest" of my cousin in her residence in a Danish castle was born in Hannover, in Germany. Her father was a businessman, her mother a woman who was frequently ill, and whose sense of hopelessness often pervaded the home. Their little girl was a sensitive, deeply religious child. Often she had meaningful experiences associated with ceremonies in the Jewish synagogue. Often she was alone, though not sad, because she experienced the presence of invisible friendly beings who played around her and kept her company.

Above all things she wanted to be a nurse. Thanks to her father, who financed her education, her hopes were fulfilled. In that work she was in her element. It gave her strength she had not realized she had. Her first experiences with nursing came in conjunction with the first world war. She cared for wounded soldiers, and in doing so she saw something that was invisible to others. She saw the auras of the wounded men in her care. She called it a "color experience."

But she herself was soon to be no longer a nurse, but a patient. She suffered with dysentery and was slow to recover. No longer able to provide care, she had to accept receiving it. She heard of a place to which she could go. There was a woman who had a nursing home, and who was said to have "healing hands." Somehow she knew that it was the right place and that this person was the one who would help her regain her strength.

Her choice was right. With the healing hands of Mrs. Bernhardt, who became very dear and important to the young nurse, she gradually was able to take on one small duty after another in the nursing home. Mrs Bernhardt, who was called Frau Maria, and her husband were also able to clarify many of her religious concepts and to answer her many questions.

When they decided to make a move to the Tyrolean Alps, Sister Rosa was invited to go with them. She was to recover fully in the fresh air and sunshine of the mountain slopes and meadows. Simple living quarters were provided for her, and she was engaged by the family as a goatherd!

It was a new life for a young person from the big city of Hannover, whose chosen occupation was nursing. But she loved it! It spoke to all that was dearest and most significant in her existence. Now there were new "color experiences", for she perceived that rocks, trees, plants flowers all had a clearly visible aura. These auras and the wonderful invisible beings that she was able to see around them spoke in new ways of things that were to become deeply meaningful in the new work that was to be hers as Sister Rosa.

That work came to an abrupt and catastrophic end with the occupation of Austria by Hitler's Third Reich. The small colony that had grown up in the proximity of the Bernhardt family was dispersed. The buildings were taken over as garrisons for Nazi troops. Sister Rosa became a refugee, who was able to flee to Denmark.

She was given refuge by a Quaker family, where my cousin Rigmor met her. The two women found many common interests, and spent many hours talking together. My cousin never forgot the essence of what her refugee friend said to her in their long talks. She wrote it down and later shared it with me. It is mine now to share with others.

"Do not forget that nothing that happens to us is accidental. The Power that creates and sustains the universe also controls human destiny. Every person has come into the world in that family, that country and that period of history in which he has the most to learn and the most to atone for. The situations we come into, the people we meet and with whom we must work, can crush us, but can also make us stronger. We must place all our strength in the service of the good. Here and now we can only see a very small part of the life pattern in which no fate is accidental or meaningless. This life is only a fragment."

It was a natural outcome of their close association and the circumstances of the Nazi occupation of Denmark that Sister Rosa was invited to come and live with my cousin in the small quarters she occupied in the Castle of Jaegerspris.

To the quiet retreat Sister Rosa came, at a time when the Nazi persecution of the Jewish people in Denmark had become more stringent, and also at a time when the presence of Nazi troops in the nearby town was extended to encompass the castle itself and its environs. The children were kept indoors; doors that had been left open were locked and precautions of many kinds were undertaken to ensure the safety of my cousin's "illegal guest." No one must be aware of her presence, since it was impossible to know which of those working in the school might be an informer.

Eventually the danger became too great. It was necessary for both of them to leave the castle and to find a safer hiding place. Many assisted them in moving from one place to another. Some who were most helpful were able in this way to extend their thanks for the healing teas or simply health advice from "Miss Fenger's nice friend." Thanks to the assistance of my cousin's father, a simple row-house was purchased on the outskirts of Copenhagen, and the two women were safely installed there.

In the constant stress and anxiety imposed by safeguarding a secret visitor both were sustained by the invaluable wisdom offered by the book that had come with Sister Rosa in her refugee baggage. It was the source of unwavering strength and support. That book was the one written by Sister Rosa's friend, Mr. Bernhardt, who had already played such an important role in her life. *In the Light of Truth* is the same book that today is the greatest treasure in my own life.

On the 5th of May 1945, the long demanding years came to an end and they saw the last of the occupation forces in Denmark. A year later, Sister Rosa was able to return to Austria. My cousin followed soon after in order to assist in the lengthy process of reconstruction and rebuilding insofar as possible the life that had been there in the Tyrolean Alps. Mr. Bernhardt, held in captivity under house arrest by the Nazis, died in 1941, but the family was able to return to their old home when the war ended.

* * * * *

Once travel to Europe was again feasible after the war, I returned to Denmark with my mother and sister. Nature was kind, and we experienced a memorable summer with fair skies and welcoming relatives The cousin who had always figured in my life had retuned from Austria, and had many things to tell. I found that she could also answer the questions of a spiritual nature to which others had not yet responded satisfactorily.

I had been a teacher, at that time, for a year, and hoped always to be a teacher. But I now felt strongly impelled to remain in Europe. My father supported the urge, and provided the funds to help make it possible. During the year that ensued there were many long talks with my cousin Rigmor and many gradually developing insights.

There was also a trip to Austria. And there I met Sister Rosa, who was now to be numbered among the many I had already encountered in my wellness adventures. Through her I would have close personal experience with an approach to healing that I had known about previously only through reading.

The Tyrolean Alps were for me a new world, and the small apartment in the simple wooden structure that I entered to meet my cousin's special friend was unlike any place I had ever been in before. I was overwhelmed at once by the fragrance of dried and drying plants, leaves, stems, roots and blossoms. It was enormously pleasant; there was something so very real about it. I wanted to stay here, to be surrounded and enveloped by the wonderful scents.

The woman to whom I was introduced was a nurse, and she went by the title afforded nurses in German speaking countries, previously in my own country as well. Sister Rosa was dressed in the simple garb of those in her profession in Germany--a plain blue dress with a high white collar, bordered with lace, and a wide, white apron. On her head was a white nurse's cap, which in time became very familiar to me, for she was never without it. The blue eyes behind the glasses observed me closely and twinkled a friendly welcome.

In this land, whose language I did not speak, it was good to know that Sister Rosa spoke Danish. I knew that, like me, she valued the book *in the Light of Truth* as her dearest possession. I had had months of time, without the unrelenting demands of work, family or telephones, to absorb its wisdom, This represented an important connection, but I knew that the book itself was mine alone. All that it transmitted spoke to me personally. It was totally mine. For each of us, from such vastly different worlds, the same was true.

Soon we were seated at the oval table under the hanging lamp in the single room that was at once sitting room, dining room, and (I learned later), also the room in which she met those who came to her for advice and help with their health problems.

On the following day, I could hardly wait to get out and see the towering mountains, the green meadows, the woodland pathways, and all the growing things that were so essential to the work of a healer. Cows grazed in the pastures, and their bells rang sweetly in my ears, and still do in my memory.

The fields and woods were brimming with health help. Everywhere there were flowers. When I tried to bring some of them back with me I soon learned that there was a wide difference between those that were nice for table decoration and those that were invaluable in teas, oils and tinctures to bring healing to those who needed Sister Rosa's help.

I watched her quietly from the adjacent room as she met with patients, asking questions as she rested her kind eyes upon them. I knew that she saw a great deal more than the physical features and the garb of the person who sat before her. She wrote on her notepad and passed the paper with the patient's name and a list of herbal names and numbers beside them to her assistant.

There was always someone as a volunteer helper, often a lady from France, to offer a hand with the wide trays of drying herbs that were kept in the attic, and to prepare them to be stored as teas, ready to be weighed or measured with other herbs in individual prescriptions for her patients.

A bag of herbs of my very own went home with me to the states, and also other bags for my parents. Sister Rosa was able to see what was needed for them when she studied the photographs that I brought for her to see.

I was always careful about how many photographs I showed her, for it was quite clear that she saw a great deal in the pictures. "He should be careful with his kidneys," she might say. Or of a child whose picture she was shown: "This one will have a difficult time." She became completely absorbed in what the photographs told her about a person. Whatever she said was purely spontaneous. Her comments came in the same way that others might say, "Oh, isn't she cute!" or "He looks like his father."

She was also closely associated, as well, with the world around her. She was ready to speak a kind word, offer praise for work well done, or to chat with neighboring farmers when she met them on the road. The folks from the farms in the vicinity all came, on her 90th birthday, some years later, to bring their congratulations and wish her well.

We knew that we should be careful not to speak of something that would entail her having to get up from the supper table to fetch a thing that was mentioned and show it to us. She was always a living example of the old saying "no sooner said than done." It was a habit worthy of emulation. Don't they say that in heaven word and deed are one?

She loved to give us pleasure. I remember her joy at sharing the box of chocolates someone had brought her. When I reminded her that she had recommended a few days before that I not indulge in chocolate at the moment, she chuckled and said, "Here, have another. After all we are not fanatics!"

When I parted from them, for my cousin was staying on after I left, my new friend gave me a warm handshake. With a look at my cousin she said firmly. "The girl will be back." And indeed I did go back, more than once to see my friend, the healer, Sister Rosa.

She is elsewhere now, beyond this earth, and the place where she lived has changed. I will not see that person or that place again. But both remain gratefully in my thoughts.

CHAPTER SEVEN

The First Modern Physician!

Paracelsus! The name still evokes a response! We know he was important--a man whose name is intimately associated with medicine. With the barest smattering of knowledge we may remember that he is called the father of modern chemistry that he dealt with alchemy and that he is credited with introducing opium and mercury into medicine.

Paracelsus stated repeatedly that sickness always comes from disobeying the natural laws. The natural laws are related to health.

Sounds like Hildegard, doesn't it? Actually, Hildegard, who talked with so many--men and women of high and low degree-- could have enjoyed a good long chat with Paracelsus. They would have agreed on so many things!

Both were devout. God was important to them. They knew that relationship with the Deity was an important aspect of health. They understood nature and recognized its importance in supplying and supporting health. Both emphasized the significance of balance in all things and the need for sensible nutrition. Both sought to restore health by natural means, so it would not be necessary to recover first from the ailment and later from the cure.

Both Hildegard and Paracelsus declared that people must learn how to become their own physicians. They would have loved to discuss the how! Yet the two could never have participated in such an enjoyable conversation ! Four centuries separated them. Paracelsus was born a year after Columbus discovered America. His mother died when he was very young and he was left with his father, a distinguished physician who became his son's first instructor. The boy was full of curiosity: he was interested in everything the world had to offer. His father's teachings were important, but he also watched the mining operations near where he lived and learned about mining and how to analyze metals. Everywhere he observed and assimilated knowledge. All his life he was quick to talk with and find out from people of every kind and station whatever they knew about and had to tell.

Of course he put in an appearance at the village school in the remote corner of Switzerland where he lived, but it did not hold his attention for long. By the time he was 14 he had set off for institutes of higher learning. By the age of 16 he was well acquainted with the current literature about alchemy. At 17 he completed his formal education with a medical degree from the University of Vienna. Soon after that he earned another medical degree from the University of Ferrara in Italy.

All told he probably attended seven universities before he had had enough of the dry scholasticism he found there. His comment regarding it has survived him: "I wonder how the high colleges manage to produce so many asses." Experience, he found, was the best teacher.

And experience was available in plenty, not only in Europe and Britain, but also in more distant places. There were opportunities to serve: he became an army surgeon in the Netherlands and Italy. Always he sought out new sources of wisdom related to the arts of alchemy and successful medical treatments. He traveled to Russia, to Arabia and Constantinople as well as to Egypt and the Holy Land. He wanted to know what others had found out and were utilizing in what he termed "the latent forces of nature"

Everywhere he was accorded recognition as a skilled physician. He became known as Paracelsus, a name he chose for himself and preferred over any one of the roster of distinguished ones with which he had been tagged at his christening. His chosen name, which meant "over or beyond Celsus," bespoke his opinion of himself as even greater than the famous first century Roman doctor who bore that name.

When he returned to Europe after his extensive travels, his students were in enthusiastic agreement about welcoming him. From far and wide they came to the lecture rooms where he taught at the University of Basel, filling them to overflowing. He taught as he wrote, not in the usual and expected Latin, but in German, the language of the people. Foremost among his writings was the renowned *Great Surgery Book*, also written in German.

Outspoken and quick-witted, doubtless arrogant at times, Paracelsus had many friends and also a number of enemies. He did not hesitate to express his disdain for anything that earned his scorn or disrespect. The authorities were shocked when he pinned on a university notice board an announcement inviting not only students, but anyone else who was interested, to attend one of his forthcoming lectures. A few years later he burned the books of Avicenna, the Arab "prince of physicians" and Galen, the famous Greek physician, in front of the University.

These provocative actions call to mind Martin Luther, whose similar actions during the same time period had provoked similar attention. Of this Paracelsus spoke as follows: "Why do you call me a medical Luther?... I leave it to Luther to defend what he says, and I will be responsible for what I say. That which you wish to Luther, you wish also to me, you wish us both in the fire."

The university faculty was indeed incensed, but the students loved him. However the number of his enemies increased, and it became necessary for him, as it was for Luther, to flee for his life, and rely upon the kindness of friends throughout central Europe to provide him with support and safe refuge. For a time he made his way from one friend to another, never staying in one place for more than a year.

His reputation was restored with the publication of his masterwork, *The Great Surgery*. For the last five years of his life he was sought out, as Hildegard had been, by crowned heads and distinguished personages throughout Europe. He became wealthy and attained even greater fame than he had known before.

His death, at the age of 48, was surrounded by unusual circumstances believed by some to have been an assassination attempt. He was buried, as had been his wish, in the graveyard of the church of St Sebastian in Salzburg. He was and is remembered as a scholar, a teacher, writer and doctor who made outstanding advances in medical science.

* * * * *

Many of those left to remember him were not among the rich and famous, but among the common people. Not only did he relate to them as friends, he respected them for the knowledge and wisdom he was able to perceive and acknowledge among them. He wrote: "The universities do not teach all things, so a doctor must seek out old wives, gypsies, sorcerers, wandering tribes, old robbers and such outlaws and take lessons from them."

From these, and from other sources, it is interesting to contemplate some of the ideas that formed the basis of the great man's thinking.

There is much of value here for our own reflection.

We must recognize with respect the importance he gave to good thoughts, good words and good deeds. They help, he said, to maintain health or to destroy it. They are among the invisible powers that we can use, for better or worse.

The "universal force" of which he spoke, he defined as being available to all, by whatever name we may call it, through prayer. Good prayer is a part of being in harmony, in balance with the laws of nature. If we disobey the natural laws relating to health, the human body will avenge itself upon us.

The universal life force comes to us from the sun, from outer space, from the growing things that we use or transform into food. Food is a medium for transmitting the life force. The energy of the life force is also present in the earth and in minerals and metals. In human beings it is present in our volition.

All things in nature are useful or benevolent in some way, Paracelsus believed. Even poison can be useful if we can discover its utility. Human beings must learn how to use the gifts of nature, and not interfere with their proper use through wrong thoughts and emotions. Therapy may consist of rightly directing or redirecting the energy of the life force everywhere around and within us.

Stress is the beginning of many ailments, he said. Mental stress can be communicated to others, even from one generation to another, or by association of human beings with others of their kind. We might reasonably surmise that Paracelsus believed in reincarnation, that he understood the effects of the law of attraction in bringing like-minded human souls together.

Any treatment that reduces tension is valid. Certain illnesses can be cured by chemical remedies; medical substances are also to be found in herbs, sometimes in combination with minerals. Nutrition is important too in maintaining or restoring health.

There is a remedy for every human ill, and everything in nature can be used in a positive and beneficial way. Visual and auditory art, accessed through our human senses, can contribute to bringing us into balance with nature. In this, painting, music, dance, theater, even architecture can play a part. These can affect significantly the type of energy force that surrounds us.

* * * * *

Paracelsus recognized the power of what is termed "magic", but he also recognized its dangers and felt that this power should be utilized only by gifted physicians, dedicated to serving not only human beings, but in perfect harmony with the laws of God and nature. However, he found it beneficial for some patients to make use of magical formulas or symbols, called talismans. They were written on paper or parchment, but might also be engraved on the surface of a gem or on metal, sometimes on the familiar medals of saints. These helped to give a positive focus to the patient's mind and attention. Paracelsus believed that they attracted the invisible energies from space to enter the magnetic field of the sick person and convey healing.

The use of talismans may have caused some persons to dismiss Paracelsus as a mystic. A greater number, however, recognized the wisdom of the metaphysical knowledge he had made his own, especially from his studies in Constantinople.

* * * * *

Wherever he went in his travels, Paracelsus would have encountered stories of the invisible folk that populate the earth everywhere. The common people whom he always chose to contact were happy to share with him their experiences with these invisibles. He understood that these experiences were not delusions or fabrications. They were real happenings. "Elementals" was the name he gave to the beings described to him.

And while there were distinct differences among the human beings he met in Europe and those in other places like Russia, Egypt and the near East, there were distinct similarities among the elementals, no matter where they were encountered.

Paracelsus, always eager to record what he learned and knew from experience, described in writing his knowledge of the elementals. They were of a different kind, he wrote, than human beings. They had no personal volition as did men; their will was totally anchored in natural law. Their activity was devoted primarily to caring for and protecting nature; In this, and in other ways, they were helpful to mankind. They were of four different kinds, related to earth, air, water and fire.

The elementals associated with earth tended and nurtured trees, plants, moss and flowers, as well as the earth itself and the rocks, stones, metals and minerals that live in the earth. These were elves, trolls and fairies, and in the case of mountains and valleys…giants.

Water nymphs populated and cared for streams, rivers, lakes and seas. Sylphs stirred and moved earthly winds and breezes and safeguarded their purity. Salamanders were active in fire, especially in volcanoes.

These elementals, he wrote, are divided into races and groups and are ruled over by kings and queens. We read of these rulers of the elementals in all the world's folklore; they share common characteristics and are known to us as gods and goddesses. Belief in these invisible beings does not conflict with orthodox religious beliefs, said Paracelsus.

Quite different in kind, however, he wrote, is a group of beings he termed "elementaries".These are not natural beings, like the elementals; they are artificial creatures brought into being by excesses of human thought and emotion. Mostly they are of a destructive nature. We would call them demons. Human energy is drained by giving support to the growth of these creatures.

The elementaries created by wrong human thought and emotion can bring harm--crime, war and also disease. But human thought and emotion can also create kindly, benign beings that contribute to the well being of good people.

*****

Ever again, in his writing, Paracelsus emphasized man's responsibility, not only with regard to our own health, but for the health of the world we live in. Man, he said, has the power to change himself. He must make good use of the life energy that is given us. He must be willing to give up bad habits that sap his strength, like overeating. He has to relinquish false beliefs and negative attitudes He must learn to respect life, to give help to those who are in need. He must engage in activities that strengthen him. In doing so he attracts life force and blessing.

To accept our responsibility is essential for every human being. It is essential for physicians who work to heal or correct the physical ills that beset us. It is essential for us when we work with physicians to regain our health. To accept our responsibility as human beings is essential for us if we are to become, as Paracelsus advised, "our own physicians."

Negative thoughts and emotions play an important part in our well being. Paracelsus understood this well. If we disobey the laws of God and nature, we will pay the price. We will reap what we may well have forgotten that we sowed.

With his vast knowledge of the multiple facets of health and healing-- chemistry, alchemy, magnetic healing, metaphysics, the effect of natural remedies, Paracelsus may also be counted among the first to understand psychosomatic therapy.

Much of what he wrote is attaining new relevance today by those physicians whose efforts are directed toward complementary and alternative medicine.

* * * * *

Any of us may hear about a remedy credited to Paracelsus, and still thankfully make use of it today. A good friend may say to you, no matter what your physical ill: "You need some Swedish Bitters."

The dark brown liquid you buy at the health food store is composed of infusions of a long list of herbs in a bit of water and alcohol. A very small amount taken in a teaspoon or used as a compress or stirred into a tea may give you effective treatment for almost any human ill or complaint. It is known and widely used by the Amish people and by those of us lucky enough to have a friend who offers good health advice.

My own experience was with gingivitis. The dentist wanted to send me to a specialist to treat my gums. I talked with my friend who said, "No, what you need is Swedish Bitters." A mouthful swooshed about over teeth and gums morning and evening was easy to use. The beneficial effect was immediately apparent to the dentist when I returned to his office some months later.

When I told this story, in a women's group I had joined, everyone there grabbed a pen or pencil and wrote down the words "Swedish Bitters." I heard later that there had been a run on the product at the local health food store.

Did Paracelsus give the formula its name, or did the name come later? We don't really know. It isn't hard to imagine that Paracelsus, with his lively interest and curiosity about all kinds of healing, came across the remedy on his travels in Scandinavia. Actually it was rediscovered a couple of centuries after Paracelsus might have discovered it, in the writings of a Swedish physician. That gentleman had inherited it as part of the family tradition. It had been put to good use. His ancestors had lived long lives, and Dr. Samst himself became 104 and died, not of some ailment or illness, but of an accident that came about when he was horseback riding. Be that as it may, it is the name of Paracelsus that endures on the Swedish Bitters label.

Not mentioned by name, but only as a "distinguished Austrian herbalist" in the same context is Maria Treben, a lady who has done much to make the ancient remedy known and correctly used.

In her book, *Health Through God's Pharmacy* she shares her knowledge and advice about the use of common herbs. She offers guidance, as well, about the proper use of Swedish Bitters.

Her own story reads indeed, as she says, "like a fairy tale". As a very young woman she was released from a Nazi concentration camp with typhoid fever. She was still extremely ill, and the doctors were unable to restore her to health. Then a neighbor came with a small bottle containing a dark, strong-smelling liquid. Along with it she passed on the transcript of writings about the strange remedy, which was said to provide treatment for all diseases.

Maria Treben thanked her neighbor and put the bottle on a shelf in her medicine chest. She could not believe that it would be of any help after all the attempts that had already been made by the doctors to make her well. But then she unexpectedly changed her mind.

A large basket of pears had to be used right away. As she got busy coring and peeling, she experienced terrible abdominal pain. What about the strange liquid her neighbor had brought her? She said it could be used externally as well as internally. Quickly she put a little on a cloth, put a plastic bag over it and tied it in place over her abdomen. She left it on all day.

She experienced a wonderful, warm feeling that gradually spread throughout her body. For the first time in many months she felt well. That single compress made her well and the terrible pain she had suffered never returned.

Gradually she developed a strong interest in herbs. With the knowledge she accumulated she was able to help many people. In her books, especially *Health Through God's Pharmacy* she offers guidance and advice to others who want to know about herbs and how to use them. She felt that she was guided by a Higher Power.

The words written in that book are like an echo of the words of Hildegard of Bingen and Paracelsus. She writes: "I endeavour to not only show you the herbs and their medicinal properties, but above all the omnipotence of a Creator in whose hands we exist."

CHAPTER EIGHT

A Revolutionary Discovery

Experience helped me to make wise choices. I was able to enjoy good health in retirement. I left Arizona, where I had cared for my elderly parents, but kept in touch and sometimes visited the extended family members who still lived there.

Two of them were victims of cancer--a niece and an in-law, who had been the wife of the young man who was my nephew. My niece, Clare, lived with her forest ranger husband in northern Arizona east of the Grand Canyon. They had a little boy. Clare and Catherine, who lived with her three boys in Tucson, shared a close and meaningful friendship.

A visit to Clare was a treat for me and for Catherine. In memory I see us all beside a mountain stream, Clare with her three-year-old, Catherine with her two youngest boys. The two women were wearing kerchiefs on their heads. Both were losing hair through the radiation and chemo they were undergoing. Clare for ovarian cancer, Catherine for lymphoma. All of that was forgotten as we enjoyed a happy day together. It was one of many good days in that memorable visit.

Later I read about Dr. William Lane's work with shark cartilage for treating cancer and talked with Clare about it. She tried in vain to find access to such treatment. Meanwhile Catherine had opted for abandoning orthodox treatment and was seeking alternative help.

In Ohio I attended a book exhibition in Cleveland. It was exciting to hear that Dr Lane was present there. I was able to speak with him moments before he took off for the airport. He was going to Japan, he said, and chuckled as he added: "They always meet me there with two limousines. I really don't know why, but they do appreciate what I have to say."

He listened closely as I told him about my two friends in Arizona. He informed me about where to procure the best shark cartilage. Then he said, "Shark cartilage, though, is no help for lymphoma. But I can tell you where to go to get reliable help". He gave me the name and telephone number of a nutritionist in Pennsylvania who was giving telephone consultations to cancer patients who wished to go the alternative or complementary route for treatment.

I was happy to part from the distinguished elderly gentleman with good wishes and with the important information in my hand.

It was a privilege to meet with the nutritionist on the telephone. She has a very fine, sensitive ability to communicate person to person with those who contact her. It was good that Clare was able to speak with her. It gave her a friendly, understanding hand across the miles in her last days here on earth. Her husband did purchase the shark cartilage for her, but it came too late. She died not long after its coming; she was not quite 37.

For Catherine, our new friend suggested a number of natural alternative remedies that I was happy to be able to help her purchase. They were good, but after some months I wondered if there might be an easier way...."Is there a single product," I asked, "that could take the place of some or all of these many products?" She hesitated for a few moments, then burst out, "Of course! – Transfer Factor!"

This was news to me, but as she told me about it, I felt that it all made sense. It made sense to Catherine too when I told her about it. Transfer Factor became her one and only remedy and treatment.

There was little else either of us could afford to provide except for basic sensible nutrition.

Approximately two years later, when she had the annual physical check up, the report read: "Cancer free."

It was good to share this news with our nutritionist friend. After we had rejoiced together over Catherine, this good person spoke the few words I will never forget: "And we remember Clare…"

* * * * *

What is Transfer Factor? Who discovered it? Perhaps we should ask first: What are transfer factors? They are not vitamins or minerals. They are not herbs of hormones. They are certainly not drugs.

Actually all of us have transfer factors in our bodies. They are tiny molecules that constitute an important part of our immune systems. As babies, if we were breast fed, we received transfer factors in the first milk (colostrum) from our mothers after we were born.

The mother's immune system is obviously more experienced than that of the newborn child, and in her colostrum the baby receives the benefit of her experience in fighting off thousands of infections. She has met and become immune to them. Her immunity is transferred to her child.

This basic knowledge is related to the discovery made by Dr. H. Sherwood Lawrence in 1949. He was studying tuberculosis and discovered that an injection from the white blood cells of a person who had developed immunity to the disease could be transferred to someone else who was not immune. The donor's immunity could be transferred to that other person. There was a molecule in the donor's system that could communicate with the immune cells in the recipient's system. Dr. Lawrence called this molecule a "transfer factor."

This was an exciting discovery that would have received more attention if it had not had to compete with the discovery of penicillin, which was attracting major interest and excitement at the time. Antibiotics were on center stage. Furthermore, the extraction and injection of transfer factor molecules were costly and time consuming.

But during that period, two scientists who were teaching at the University of South Carolina made another important discovery. They found that transfer factors were not "species specific." In other words human beings could benefit from the colostrum extracted from animals, specifically cows. The colostrum could be extracted, dried and put in capsules. The extraction process was patented by the two researchers in 1989.

The patent remained obscure and unknown until another man ran across the information in the pursuit of knowledge related to his own health problem. David Lisonbee had been made aware of the importance of nutrition by his mother. She wrote books about nutrition; she saw to it that her son ate properly and that he got his vitamins. He followed her good advice on into adulthood. Nevertheless. in maturity he battled a constantly recurring upper respiratory infection.

For years he sought out products and programs related to supporting the immune system. He understood the importance of vitamins, minerals, herbs, and healthy foods. He did not need any more information about those subjects.

Then, in an obscure reference to a patent for the extraction of molecules called "transfer factors" he knew that he had at last found what he had been seeking for such a long time.

The answer was related to the body's own immune system. Nobody can be healthy unless he has a strong immune system. The little-known molecule that could be extracted from the colostrum of cows and taken orally was his answer! It must have felt to him like finding the gold at the end of the rainbow!

The knowledge had to be shared. With his wife, David Lisonbee secured the rights to the only existing patent for the extraction of transfer factor, Subsequently he realized that the molecule was present and could be extracted from avian sources as well—from chicken eggs!

Together, the Lisonbees soon became convinced that the products containing transfer factor must be made known to the world. But creating a company is not a thing "no sooner said than done." It involved personal expenditures and total commitment on their part.

It meant thoughtful planning and carefully weighed decisions.

Offers to make transfer factor available commercially came from pharmaceutical companies, franchises and department stores. All were ultimately refused. It was felt that the most responsible way to deal with this wonderful new product was to make it available only through multi-level marketing. Person to person contact would also make it possible to refer people to knowledgeable physicians if that was desired or advised.

The company established by the Lisonbees was called 4LifeResearch. The product called Transfer Factor was made available to the public about a year before it was recommended for my friend Catherine, as told at the beginning of this chapter. A series of scientific discoveries and the dedicated, unselfish efforts of people she had never met brought her the health miracle for which she had hoped.

Decades of worldwide independent study had preceded the establishment of 4LifeResearch. Over 3000 clinical studies and papers had been published about transfer factors. The International Transfer Factor Society was established in 1999 to "promote, stimulate and coordinate the exchange of ideas related to studies of Transfer Factor and other immunoregulators." It does not endorse any commercial products.

Studies have demonstrated transfer factors to be effective and safe. There have been no reported side effects. All over the world independent researchers, clinicians, universities and hospitals have tested and made use of transfer factors.

The products offered by 4LifeResearch are called simply Transfer Factor. One of its products has been shown to increase the effectiveness of our immune system by 437%. This was reported by studies in Russia. 4Life Transfer Factor products have become the first supplements approved in Russia for use by doctors in hospitals throughout that country.

In the United States 4Life products are listed in the *Physician's Desk Reference for Nonprescription Drugs and Dietary Supplements.* This is a statement from that reference: "Transfer factors educate the immune system to recognize self from non-self, thus supporting healthy immune system function. Because they instruct the immune system to act appropriately, transfer factors are effective in supporting normal inflammation response in the body, a key to healthy body system function."

Transfer factors don't directly fight disease, but they help to keep us healthy so we're not likely to catch diseases. Transfer factors regulate our immune system, our overall health. They even affect premature aging. If you have a healthy immune system you are more likely to stay healthy, no matter whether you're young or old.

As a senior I always keep Transfer Factor on hand for the moments when I feel as though I might be "catching something." I also protect myself with the products especially beneficial for the cardiovascular system and the brain These are important products for older people to know about and use.

The company has a number of products that have transfer factor combined with other natural compounds directed toward affecting specific conditions. Scientists working with 4LifeResearch have developed a number of new patents over time.

I had anticipated the pleasure of sharing my new knowledge with my veterinarian. I was disappointed. He knew all about it! Actually the first use of the product in the animal world was with horses. Since then, dogs and other animals have likewise benefited from Transfer Factor.

Some people discover for themselves how it may benefit them to have an immune system that really supports and protects their health. One friend no longer dreads the approach of spring. He can finally enjoy it, since he's no longer bothered with allergies.

Another friend was prepared to battle melanoma after it was diagnosed. Encouraged to take Transfer Factor before, during and after surgery he was happy to hear the results. Scans all over his body revealed no cancer. He felt that a strong immune system contributed to this good report.

I'll let another friend speak for herself:

"To build and regulate the immune system, the main thing I have found is TRANSFER FACTOR. It is highly praised among many, including cancer patients. It is powerful yet safe. My motto is "first do no harm" and I believe Transfer Factor fits that description. It has helped me in a big way with my leukemia!!!"

* * * * *

As infants we received colostrum from our mothers. It gave us a good start before our immune systems were fully developed. The knowledge that we could continue to receive powerful immune support throughout our lives was a revolutionary discovery. Since It appeared at about the same time as penicillin it did not receive early recognition. For a while penicillin was on center stage. But eventually scientists and physicians all over the world have given it their attention. They have been working with it for over 60 years, resulting in thousands of research papers and independent studies.

Creating a product from cow colostrum and eggs that was pure and safe for human beings was not easy, but it happened and finally the product was patented and made available commercially. I was referred to the most reliable company from which to purchase transfer factor, 4LifeResearch. It has been good to see this company thrive and also respond swiftly to human need with voluntary donations of its products for victims of catastrophe and disaster all over the world.

The identification and isolation of transfer factor molecules has been called the greatest discovery in preventive medicine since penicillin. These vital molecules don't just regulate the immune system; they help to regulate and preserve our body's entire health.

As we acknowledge the presence of hazards to our health in the food we eat, the air we breathe, the water we drink, it becomes increasingly important for us to seek and recognize dependable health help. Big business knows how to market products that purport to supply our needs. Personal experience has taught me which companies and which products can be trusted.

*****

My niece Catherine and I have cooperated in creating the company called THE SHINING SWAN. Its website www.theshiningswan.com has links to three companies. One of them is 4LifeResearch. Transfer Factor products can be viewed there and purchased at wholesale prices. New articles are added from time to time to those appearing on the site. Visitors to the site who sign in are automatically eligible for inclusion in periodic drawings. Prizes are awarded, including Transfer Factor products.

CHAPTER NINE

Health Help from the Past in New Hands

A friend introduced me to a wonderful source of health and healing.

Long, long ago it was a luxury, available only to royalty and to those who had a great deal of money. Grave robbers chose it when they had a chance, in preference to gold. It was made use of in religious practices and ceremonies. These rare and wonderful substances, accessible in centuries past only to a special few, can now be had by all of us just plain folks—people like you and me.

These incredible products are called essential oils. As children we heard about frankincense and myrrh. We knew that those things were special, since they were among the gifts brought to the Christ child. But we would never have dreamed that they were called essential oils. Oils? What kind of gift was that? Sure, we knew about oils. There was cod liver oil—who would want that for a present? And Castor Oil—yuck! Oils for cooking, oils for cleaning....What good would they be to a wonderful little baby?

History tells us that these were indeed wonderful gifts. Along with other precious treasures they were placed in the tombs of the Egyptian Pharaohs. They were known and revered by healers.

Frankincense! It is mentioned in one of the oldest known medical records, the Ebers Papyrus, dating from sixteen centuries before Christ was born. In that document it is said to be "used to treat every conceivable ill known to man."

Oh yes, little Babe, who favored this earth by coming here, we would have you protected from every possible disease. That indeed is a gift fit for a king!

And myrrh? There it is, along with frankincense, in that ancient Egyptian papyrus, And there it is again, in many Bible references.

It was said to be especially effective for skin conditions.

A fitting gift for the feet of Him who would travel many rough miles on foot with his disciples!

Myrrh was highly regarded by our friend Hildegard of Bingen. Surely Paracelsus discussed its multiple uses with those who practiced medicine in Turkey and the European countries he visited.

Yes, oh yes, this too belonged among the gifts brought by kings to honor the newly-born King!

* * * * *

What are these marvelous substances called essential oils ? How come they were so expensive? Were they hard to get? How did people get them?

Our very first encounter with an essential oil tells us that it is not like the oils with which we have been familiar. It isn't greasy. It has a very pleasant fragrance. It's different.

It is a liquid that has been part of the very essence of the life form from which it came We are told that it may be composed of hundreds of chemical compounds. And the drop of essential oil that we hold on a finger tip is extremely powerful!

It is very powerful because it wasn't derived from just a single plant, flower, seed, or root. The essence of hundreds of plants— from their flowers, their stems, roots or seeds--had to be extracted to yield the one drop of essential oil we hold on a finger tip.

This extraction was no easy matter. We know that it may have been done in ancient times by soaking petals and other plant parts in goose fat and then separating the oil from the fat, or by using boiling water, or by passing steam through plant parts to separate the oil from them. Needless to say, practice and skill were required for success. Experts worked for long hours to perfect the skill. It was not work for amateurs.

Modern technology has simplified the extraction process and made it possible to produce vast quantities of essential oil. But we can also begin to understand that careful control is required to guarantee the purity of the oil that is produced. And it is also not difficult to see how easily the essential oil may be adulterated and altered by the addition of other untrustworthy components. People have learned how to manufacture a product that is loved as perfume, but that has no beneficial health effects.

This is why standards have been developed to differentiate between what are termed "therapeutic grade essential oils" and others that are of inferior quality. France has developed measurements for these quality oils called the AFNOR scale. It is the international "gold standard" for genuine therapeutic grade essential oils.

Much important work with essential oils has been carried out in France. It was in France that a dramatic episode involving essential oil took place. A scientist was critically burned in a laboratory experiment. He plunged his flaming arm into what he assumed to be a vat of pure water. He was mistaken; the vat contained lavender oil.

To his amazement the terrible burns on his arm began to heal the very next day.

As a result of this event French doctors in the first World War began to use essential oils for wound healing and as an antibacterial agent. In World War II It was also a French doctor who made use of essential oils with surprising positive results. They were also found to be antiviral and antifungal.

In the United States there was not much work done with essential oils. It was basically confined to healers called aromatherapists whose oils came from distant lands and faraway places. Little or no research had been conducted with essential oils. Along with France, you would have to travel to Mexico, Turkey, Egypt, or Israel to seek out the experts in the field.

And it was to those places that a young American from Idaho traveled to find out more about essential oils. Gary Young had gone with his father to Canada, where he planned to dedicate his life to logging and ranching. His plans were drastically altered by an accident in which he was seriously injured. Despite months of specialized care he left the hospital in a wheelchair with the pronouncement that he could not be expected to walk again.

Discouraged and depressed, the young man at first gave little attention to those who came to encourage and advise him. But someone mentioned essential oils. His subsequent research brought the unexpected cure and sparked a lively interest that led him to those places where he could learn more about the oils that had been of such great personal importance to him.

Gary D. Young has become one of the world's outstanding researchers with essential oils. He has helped to establish standards of excellence for planting, growing and distilling oils not only in his native Utah, but also in France and Ecuador His research has led him to the discovery of plants previously unrecognized for their healing powers. Ever active, he has created oil blends that have been proven to be of significant benefit to animals as well as to human beings. He has shared his knowledge in lectures and workshops all over the world.

In recent years he has been excited to find plants for health and healing in Ecuador. Sometimes when he inquired about the name of a plant he was told that it was "just a weed." He discovered extraordinary plants previously unknown even to the natives there. He now spends half of the year in that country, with his wife and two young boys. He is helping to establish a modern oil distillery in Ecuador, and a University department in that country dedicated solely to essential oils.

In the United States he founded and is still president of the company called Young Living, in which his wife also plays an active role. The essential oils produced by Young Living are tested in independent laboratories by chemists licensed to test therapeutic grade essential oils. They must conform to international AFNOR standards.

Plants are sent to Young Living's modern distilleries from abroad; others are grown in this country. It must be a beautiful experience to see and to inhale the fantastic fragrance of the extensive fields of lavender grown by the company in Utah! Plants grown by Young Living must pass the same strict testing procedures applied to the raw materials as well as to the essential oils that are produced.

Recognized as the world's outstanding researcher in essential oils, Dr. Gary Young also participates in their production. One of his favorite activities is the annual winter balsam harvest, an exciting event in which volunteers are invited to participate. Many have learned to rejoice in the benefits of balsam essential oil.

Thanks to my friend, who discovered Young Living, I too have learned to enjoy many of the essential oils produced by this extraordinary company.

From my friend I heard about the ones she liked best. The literature invited me to try others. Familiar names were tempting: lavender and peppermint, lemon and geranium. There were many others. With a gasp I recognized another name--frankincense ! I could hold in my hands, for my own use, the same special oil that had been brought as a gift to the Christ child! It was a bit pricey for me, but there were others I could well afford.

Where to begin? I was told that the "Essential 7 Kit" was a good place to start. And there were the ones that had tempted me in the listing: peppermint, lavender, lemon. The scent of them was wonderful when they came, and I soon learned how to use them and what they were good for.

The others in the set were all oil blends, whose names provided hints about how they would prove useful. There was Purification, whose fresh cleansing scent was welcome in the dryer and the linens and other laundry that came from there, PanAway banished much physical discomfort. Peace and Calming fulfilled its name at times of stress and tension, Joy I always wanted to couple with moments of feeling especially uplifted.

My first experiences with these oils were only a beginning of explorations into their multiple uses.

Of course I had to learn the various ways of using the essential oils. It is natural, right away, to want to smell them. Actually inhaling essential oils can trigger positive responses in the body. And there are ways to increase these responses. The right kind of diffuser that disperses a fine mist of oil into the air without heating it, which could damage the oil, is a good thing to have. The fine vapor can ward off disease and strengthen and invigorate the body. A similar effect can be achieved by placing a cloth with a few drops of oil in front of a humidifier. Sometimes the effect we want to achieve can be had by putting a few drops of oil in a bowl of steaming water, covering your head and the bowl with a towel and inhaling deeply.

Another easy way to use the oils is by putting them directly on the skin, especially on the feet. Some essential oils like lavender are wonderful in our bath water, but the addition of Epsom salts with the oil will ensure that it mixes with the bath water and doesn't just float on top of it.

Some very potent oils must be diluted with a pure mixing oil, available from the company, or with pure olive oil, for instance. The literature that is sent with the oils we order tells which oils can be used directly on the skin, and which should be diluted. It also tells which oils can be diffused. Like other users, I had to learn to respect the strength and power of the oils.

One of my favorite oils is <u>Thieves</u>. There is an interesting story behind the unusual name. During the 15th Century England was ravaged by a terrible plague. The dead and dying were everywhere, and so were the thieves who busied themselves with robbing these helpless victims wherever they could. These unscrupulous individuals seemed to be immune to the terrible disease with which they were in constant contact. They never got sick!

Why not? This was the question that haunted Gary Young. It gave him no peace until he could find the answer. What was it that these men back in the middle ages had or did that kept them protected from infection? The answer was surely to be found in books or other written records. For weeks on end Gary Young was a regular visitor to the libraries in the great city of London.

Slowly the story emerged: the men were employed on vessels that brought exotic products from distant shores to England. Once apprehended, they consented to divulge the combination of oils, herbs and spices they rubbed on themselves for protection from disease.

The American visitor carefully recorded the names that would become part of an important blend of essential oils. Together they had tremendous power to fight and kill microorganisms. Their names are on the little bottle that I and so many others have found to be significant time after time when others around us succumbed to something that was "going around." Like the thieves of yore, we can be protected by a precious blend containing Clove, Lemon, Cinnamon Bark, Eucalyptus Radiata and Rosemary.

Because the feet are especially receptive to the benefits of essential oils we can apply a few drops of Thieves essential oil on our feet and enjoy immunity in a way that nobody needs to know about. We can feel safe from exposure to infection in crowded places like buses and planes, in schools and shopping malls. I like to have Thieves lozenges In my purse for easy, extra protection if people are sneezing or coughing around me.

Of course anybody who discovers essential oils has a favorite or two. My friend is devoted to Melrose, which you dilute with one part vegetable oil. She has had wonderful experiences with quick healing of cuts, scrapes, burns and bruises Melrose is a blend of essential oils that is especially effective in regenerating damaged tissue and reducing inflammation.

My own favorite is peppermint. A drop or two on the temples and forehead can banish a headache or make you more alert. I gave some to an oil truck driver who was concerned about falling asleep at the wheel. "Try this, "I told him. "A few drops on your forehead may help you as much as a cup of coffee." I diffuse some peppermint oil if I start getting drowsy over computer tasks. The same oil, in dilution, I have found to be helpful in dealing with skin conditions.

Actually, researchers at the university of Cincinnati found that inhaling peppermint oil increased mental accuracy in students by 28 percent.

Lavender is probably the most-often selected favorite. Everybody loves its fragrance, which is calming and relaxing. It's good for insect bites, burns and cuts. It can help you sleep better, and at the same time it has also been shown to improve mental acuity and concentration when it is diffused.

People love to exchange experiences with essential oils and of course we love to read testimonials. A good place to do this is on www.oil-testimonials.com. You can sign up to read the 50 latest testimonials, search for entries concerning a subject you want to read about, or enter your own experience with a favorite essential oil.

This is where to share what you know, or what you want to know.

I've found helpful information there about allergies, gum problems, insomnia and lots of others. Those who register there will subsequently be informed when new entries are posted about subjects in which they are especially interested.

Essential oils have become an important part of my life. I don't want to be without my small bottles of Lavender, Peppermint, Purification, Lemon, Thieves, Aroma Life and others. And I'm happy to have found the company Young Living. It has attained international recognition for its production of the highest quality therapeutic grade essential oils.

I understand how important it is to use pure oils, unadulterated by anything at all on the long line that begins in the field or the natural setting. Careful selection and use of the purest raw materials is of critical importance. Scrupulous distilling and constant quality testing in the development of top quality products insures users of dependable health support and protection.

I understand why clinics and universities make use of Young Living's essential oils in research. And why these are the oils that are becoming increasingly known by physicians –the ones that are being recommended by complementary doctors everywhere.

I realize that Young Living essential oils can address both physical and emotional needs. In our own family we have had very happy experiences with their use for animals. We have learned that animals generally respond to essential oils in much the same way that humans do. Exciting chapters are being added all over the world to the long, long history of essential oils.

The Essential Oils Desk Reference is a comprehensive volume that I have constantly returned to for information about the history and use of essential oils, and for specific information about those available from Young Living. A less expensive volume that is also informative and helpful is *Quick Reference Guide for using Essential Oils.*

My niece, Catherine Webner, and I have cooperated in setting up a website featuring three other sites as links. We invite you to visit http://www.theshiningswan.com, where the Young Living website is easy to access. Over time interesting articles will be added to those already available there. The names of those who sign in are automatically entered in drawings for special prizes, including essential oils.

CHAPTER TEN

Healing at Our Fingertips

I came across Reflexology, a totally new healing modality to me, a number of years ago. I was introduced to a lady who was practicing this method with good results. When I learned that she was able to help people with all kinds of problems by just working on their feet, I was naturally interested. What could be simpler and safer than that?

What did she do and how did she do it?

I wanted to learn more about reflexology. Is it a new discovery? How does it work? I remembered that Jesus had washed the feet of his disciples. That was a beautiful act of symbolic significance. The disciples interpreted it in terms of humility, an example to guide them in performing unselfish acts for others. It has been variously interpreted as having still deeper significance. However it is interpreted, the act performed by Jesus surely demonstrated that feet are important.

With our feet we contact the earth, our native soil and planet. How well we stand and walk on our feet is important to our overall well-being. Our feet support the weight of our body--actually no small accomplishment. I read that Leonardo da Vinci had called the human foot a masterpiece of engineering and a work of art.

But it was obvious that reflexology was something more than that. The new person in my life, who became my friend, was working with people's feet to provide them with help for healing. My hunch was that other people, in other times and places, had likewise practiced this healing art.

I was not wrong. An Egyptian pictograph dating from around 2500 B.C. shows two men working on the feet of two others, who are obviously patients.

Some say that reflexology began even before that in China. The Incas are said to have practiced a form of foot reflex therapy. From them it was passed on to American Indians.

How and when it may have come to native Americans, it is quite certain that it is practiced today by the Cherokee Indians and has been done so for many generations. By them it is considered to be an important healing art. The contact of our feet with the earth, they say, is important, since it puts us in touch with the energies flowing through the earth.

In the 14th century a form of reflexology was known and practiced in Europe by the common people as well as by those who treated royalty and the aristocracy.

What became known initially as Zone Therapy was first called Head's Zones, since it was derived from neurological studies carried out in the 1890's in England by Sir Henry Head. He discovered that certain zones on the skin reacted to pressure when an organ connected by nerves to this skin area was diseased. He defined specific zones and their interconnections.

At the same time a great deal of practical work was conducted in Russia. In that country reflexology was related to the theory of conditioned reflexes--that there is a simple and direct connection between a stimulus and a response. This began with psychological studies and proceeded to physical applications. So It was in Russia that reflexology was first recognized as an effective complement to traditional medicine.

In Germany massage was applied to reflex zones, as was also the case in our own country. Here in the United States Dr. Joseph Shelby Riley was making use of the knowledge about zone therapy taught by his predecessors. The reflex zones of the feet were identified but not given special attention in his practice. Eunice Ingham, who was one of his assistants, realized the major importance of the feet and began to write her own books about reflexology.

She understood how sensitive the feet are and began to target them especially in her work. She charted the zones on the feet and their relationship to the rest of the anatomy. Eunice Ingham has been called the "mother of modern reflexology." Her book, *Stories the Feet Can Tell*, tells how she was introduced to "zone therapy", which was based on the understanding that there are ten zones in the body, and that all the organs and glands lie on one or several of the zones. Each finger and toe goes to one of the zones. Through studying these zones and practicing on the feet, Eunice Ingham developed a method and thereby pioneered reflexology with great success.

It was through her book, "*Stories the Feet Can Tell*" that my friend Renate was first introduced to reflexology. In the 1980's, when I met her, she was practicing reflexology with great personal satisfaction and providing significant help to her family and others who came to her for assistance in resolving their health problems.

Eunice Ingham was able to help many people in her flourishing practice. Eventually, though, she realized that she couldn't help everyone who was in pain and was looking for a practitioner like herself. So she began giving seminars, teaching others this wonderful method.

A nephew, who had become her "guinea pig" and had benefited a great deal from her treatments, was very interested in what she was doing. He joined her in presenting the seminars. When she retired he continued the work, teaching people to help others with reflexology, not only in the United States, but all over the world. Soon he had to teach others to conduct the training seminars. They are still being taught in our country every spring and fall in many of our major cities.

This man is Dwight Byers, who has inspired many with his knowledge and enthusiasm, and who has also written his own book about reflexology.

Renate, who had been introduced to these fascinating books, and who became a certified reflexologist, also became my good friend. She had begun by sending in the card included in the book to declare her desire to attend a seminar and learn all about reflexology. Now, some 30 years and many seminars later she is still practicing part-time, even though she is now in her seventies.

She has continued her education in reflexology, and has taken several seminars with Dwight Byers. About him she says, "He always seemed extremely knowledgeable, energetic, almost driven to spread the message about this wonderful, effective and safe healing modality. I always came away from the seminars with renewed focus, new knowledge and determination to do the best I could to help people feel better and find relief from many aches and pains."

Her practice over these years was mostly part-time while raising a family of six children. The children always loved having their feet worked on by their mom, even if a spot was sometimes tender when something was out of kilter. They were happy when their aches and pains were relieved.

Even after they grew up, they always looked forward to the chance to have a foot reflex session. Many headaches, neck aches, backaches and cramps have been relieved with just one or two sessions. And now the many grandchildren stick out their little or big feet in hopes of getting the same treatment. It's a treat!

People say that reflexology makes them feel good. That is because it is a holistic healing technique. That means it treats the whole person, not just the body, but also the mind and spirit. Reflexology makes us feel good because it reduces tension and helps us to relax. With this kind of equilibrium we cooperate with the practitioner and are more open to healing.

Science has proved that healing takes place because the reflex points familiar to reflexologists relay energy along meridian lines to specific places in the body. Stimulation of the reflex points has also been shown to produce chemicals that have a calming effect.

Many people have experienced the relief and satisfaction of being able to deal with everyday problems like headaches and many others through the guidance provided by books of instruction like *Body Reflexology* by Mildred Carter and Tammy Weber. Learning to give attention to slight twinges of pain can help us to avoid things that might well develop into more serious problems.

It's nice to learn that animals too can benefit from reflexology.

It's an easy step from petting your dog to gently searching out a sore point on his paws and exerting pressure to help our furry friend over some physical distress.

As for me, I am thankful to experience this positive effect and to have a friend who can help me through specific aches and pains and offer me the benefits of this wonderful healing art. I know it to be one of the many gifts that keeps me feeling fit, well into my eighties.

* * * * *

Like Eunice Ingham, my friend Renate has wonderful stories to tell. I've asked her to share some of them in this book.

When Eddy came to me for a reflexology session, he was working for a big firm. Besides driving a big semi truck, his job included loading and unloading heavy shipments. All in all he worked for 16 or more hours a day. That owner had a special permit that allowed him to make use of his employees in this way.

Eddy had not only NO time for his family or himself, but was always in pain, extremely tired and had headaches every day that were like migraines. He had already been working in this way for 2 to 3 years.

When he slept he snored, and according to his wife he stopped breathing for long periods of time. If that wasn't enough to deal with, his constant colds certainly made his life almost unbearable.

Finally he took time off to see a doctor, who referred him to a sleep clinic in Columbus. The tests showed that he stopped breathing up to 4 minutes at a time, many times in the night. The diagnosis: sleep apnea.

He was given an appointment to be fitted with a C-pap machine, three weeks later. His grandmother, who knew about my work as a reflexologist, called me and asked if I would please work on him to see if I could be of help. I said I would certainly try, although I had never had anyone with that condition. Pleadingly she said: "We only have 3 <u>weeks</u>."

That is how I met Eddy and started working on him right away. His response to reflexology was nothing short of amazing.

After the first session he slept all night for three nights in a row. Headaches were gone! All the other symptoms just disappeared in a short time.

After six sessions he told me that the lump was gone. 'What lump?' I asked. 'The lump that was below the lowest rib, the right side toward the center, about the size of a golf ball.'

While he was at the sleep clinic the first time, he told the medics about it, and they told him it was 'from the sleep apnea.' Like the other symptoms, it just went away. I was so excited for him!

He had decided not to even bother to go back to the doctor for his appointment to be fitted for the C-pap. But I wanted him to keep his appointment and tell the doctor himself. Maybe others would benefit from all this. So grudgingly, he took time off from work and went to the scheduled appointment.

When the doctor came in Eddy asked him if the machine would be ordered for him specifically. The doctor said yes. Eddy told him not to order it because he no longer needed it.

The doctor's response was 'Fine' And he walked out.

* * * * *

When Glenn, Eddy's uncle, found out how I had helped him with the sleep apnea, he made an appointment with me in the hope that I could help him too. He was 67 at the time. A doctor in Florida had diagnosed him with the same condition that Eddy had and had urged him to have a C-pap, but Glenn refused. He had known some who had that device and had heard from others that were using one. It is very cumbersome and disruptive to the spouse, to say the least. Most move to another room for the night, if they have that luxury. In any case they all despised the apparatus and wished they didn't have to use it. Being older and heavier than Eddy made him wonder if I would be able to help him as quickly as I did his nephew, or at all. As for me I couldn't promise anything.

It was quite exciting to both of us when he responded almost as quickly as Eddy had. Obviously age or weight had no bearing on it.

When I talked with Eddy to get his approval for the article about him, he said he is doing fine and has lost some weight. He also knows who to come to if he should have problems again.

* * * * *

Let me tell you about John. He was one of the oil well tenders in our area. In the morning when Larry, my husband, was outside starting with the farm work, John was starting his day by making his rounds from well to well and he'd stop and talk to Larry for a little while.

One morning he told Larry that he was in excruciating pain with the sciatica on his left leg and hip. He'd been doctoring for it, but nothing seemed to help. It had just been getting worse and worse. He could hardly get in and out of the truck, which he had to do regularly.

Larry felt sorry for him and told him that I would probably be able to help him. When I talked to him, I asked if he could come three times a week, at 8 o'clock in the morning before he started his rounds. He heartily agreed.

Esther E. Hansen

The first time he came I had him fill out a "Client History" form. When I saw that he was a diabetic, I asked him if he tested his blood sugar every day. He said, 'No, only when I go to the doctor.' So I told him that when he came to me for reflexology sessions, he'd have to test every day. So the very next day he tested his blood first thing in the morning.

He was surprised when he couldn't find a reading on it. Baffled, he called his sister who is also a diabetic. She said, "Come on over and we'll test with mine" But the result was the same. She hurried to get the book and see what that meant. It meant that the sugar was off the chart. She told him to eat nothing but meat until it came down. And it did.

John surmised that the pain reliever and muscle relaxant the doctor had him on must have driven up his sugar. He had never had this problem before. Good thing he stopped the medication when he did!

So not only was I trying to help him with his sciatica, but I also wanted to work on his pancreas reflex, on the feet, in hopes of helping his sugar metabolism. As already mentioned earlier in this article, every part of the body is represented in the feet, as well as the hands. So working on these reflexes, we can indirectly work on every part of the body and improve its function without doing harm. That is what impressed me so much about reflexology. Doing this for over 30 years, I was again and again surprised how quickly the body responded to this indirect stimulation.

So it was also with John. He came faithfully, in spite of the discomfort he had to endure. But the reward was not far behind. After every session the sciatica pain, as well as the discomfort in his reflexes, was less and less until he was his own happy self again.

The pancreas was responding favorably too and the pain in the reflex showed less intensity with every session. When we started out his pain response was a 4 (intolerable) and by the time he was transferred to another work area, it was a 1 (only slight discomfort). His sugar readings came down into a fairly normal level and he and his wife were overjoyed. His doctor was pleased too and kept him on the same low level of medication. We spread out the sessions to just one or two a month.

Several months later he was transferred to another area and I didn't see him any more.

Many months later I called him to find out how he was getting along. Sadly, I heard that they had had a hard time keeping his sugar down and the doctor had increased his medication. But I was happy to hear that his sciatica had not reared its ugly head again since then.

* * * * *

The Ohio Association of Reflexology usually has a booth at the annual Light Expo in Columbus, Ohio.

Once I worked a shift there and a lady from a booth nearby came over to try out what we were doing.

She was very impressed and enjoyed having her feet worked on. She asked all kinds of questions about how this works and I told her about some testimonials.

My newest success, I told her, was with sleep apnea. Her eyes got big and she told me that her husband, a medical doctor, has had that problem for quite some time.

After I was finished with her, she sent him over right away. After getting comfortable in my chair and, (quite interested in what I was doing), he told me that he has had two surgeries for the "sleep apnea" and it didn't help at all.

I explained to him that the problem wasn't inside the throat, where they did the surgery, but was coming from the neck. I just followed the sore spots on the feet, which pointed to the neck area. Once I concentrated on these reflexes and worked out the sore spots, the problem went away very quickly.

Esther E. Hansen

I asked him this very important question, that has bothered me for a long time, 'Why are doctors not looking at the cervical spine, when they can't find any other reason for the problem? Why do surgery inside a healthy throat, and do it a <u>second time</u>, when the first one was unsuccessful????'

After doing reflexology for over 30 years and having experienced amazing results, I still wonder why doctors still don't look at the spine for unexplained causes, knowing that the nerves to <u>all</u> parts of the body come out of the spine somewhere!!!!'

One of my former clients came back to see me recently, after 5 years, to have some reflexology sessions again. The reason she came to me before was that she had been suffering, for several months, with terrible headaches. Whatever drugs the doctors gave her; nothing seemed to work. It may have given her some relief for a while but as soon as she stopped the pills the headache was back. So it went from one medication to another, until someone suggested to maybe try reflexology. She was at a point of trying almost anything in the hope of getting relief.

Since I didn't remember what her reason was for coming to me the first time, she excitedly filled me in on what had happened. After filling out a client report and telling me her pain filled story, I got her settled in and started working on her feet. After the one hour session, and according to my findings; I had recommended for her to come 6 times, no longer than 1 week apart, in the hopes of giving her lasting relief. And that is what she did. The headaches were gone and never came back

I was happy to see her again and hear the story. I sincerely hope that I will be as successful as before, in helping her.

Chapter Eleven

The Touch of Healing

It was thanks to my chiropractor and the special testing he made available that I was diagnosed with osteoporosis. My mother had suffered from the disease; I had watched her twice break a hip and then fall, each time breaking a hip before the fall. I had seen her living with other fractures.

I felt that the body awareness I had assimilated from my gifted friend Mascha would serve me well now. It would be a valuable protection and precaution in dealing with any evidence of disease I might encounter. I was alert to the need for natural supplements that would support my bodily needs.

I visited the chiropractor from time to time and respected his advice. Once he expressed concern about my left leg and referred me to a practitioner who worked with modalities that were new to me. Surprise! I told him that I had just met in his waiting room the person to whom he had referred me! We had experienced a pleasant chat together.

I was happy to meet Patricia Csaba again as a patient. Ultimately we became good friends.

I learned to value the gentle non-invasive "touch of healing" associated with the energy work practiced by my new friend. Was it touch? Sometimes she worked above the body. Always I left the treatments feeling strong, well and somehow uplifted.

* * * * *

Energy… I thought about it, wondered about it…It's a very long time in my rather long life since the science classes I lived through in high school and college. They left me mystified and mostly ignorant insofar as providing permanent wisdom was concerned.

I knew that Einstein had brought forth an understanding that must be honored and respected. It was about energy. And the formula, dutifully learned and rendered on exams as a student, meant that energy is the same as mass. Now, all these years later, I tried to make sense of that.

Okay, mass is absolutely everything in and around us. Mass means things that we can see, hear, smell, feel. It is the chair in which I am comfortably seated, the fire burning in my wood stove, the little dog curled up beside me...all living things, including me! It is the book I am reading, the fields outside my window. The window itself!

But there are multiple things less visible than these: the sunbeams that come slanting through the window panes, the wind that rattles the door on my porch, the bang I hear as it is blown loose and swings open. These too are forms of energy.

Lately, in accessing messages, advertising, information and much besides, I have become aware of the vast, unfathomable reaches of the internet. Invisible, all those forms of energy fill the air, which is also energy, in and around me.

The words that I write are visible to my eye, they are perceptible to my ear when I speak. The thoughts that engendered them are invisible, but they are also forms of energy.

My thoughts contain emotions that are or become new forms of energy. They express joy or sorrow. I approve or criticize, I love or hate. Science has even measured thoughts, along with heat and light and other kinds of energy that are invisible.

These simple basic facts, verified today by quantum physics, provide perhaps an introduction to the extensive world of "energy therapies."

A great deal more is implied and incorporated in the word "energy" than may be achieved as a "physical burst of strength" derived from an exercise, or a bowl of fortified vitamin-enriched breakfast cereal.

In ancient times healers knew and understood energy. They gave various names to their basic knowledge, and utilized it in multiple ways. In Japan the knowledge was shaped into what became the art ot Jin Shin Jyutsu, one of the modalities known and practiced by my friend Patricia.

Jin Shin Jyutsu came to the United States in modern times thanks to a Japanese American woman who went to Japan from Seattle, Washington, where she was born, expecting to enter a Japanese University. Her plans were to become a translator and to study diplomacy. She longed to overcome the prejudice against the Japanese in the States, resulting from the Second World War and the unfortunate treatment of the Japanese in our country.

Once in Japan, however, her plans were dramatically altered. She met a man who had been actively involved in the recent revival of the ancient art of Jin Shin Jyutsu and had become its major proponent in Japan. She met him at the home of a mutual friend. Naturally he spoke with enthusiasm of the new life it had opened to him. He expressed his hopes for the use of Jin Shin Jyutsu as a significant help to human health. When he asked her if she would like to study with him she spontaneously answered, "Yes."

Shortly after this voluntary commitment she became seriously ill for the first time ever in her life. The man who had become her teacher now also became her healer. She not only became well, she remained in Japan for 12 years, studying with Jiro Murai.

Mary Burmeister returned to the United States. She was never ill again. She became the world's foremost teacher of Jin Shin Jyutsu.

At teaching centers all over our country, American practitioners have learned to practice the ancient art. The principal center is located in Scottsdale, Arizona. Jin Shin Jyutsu is one of the modalities used by my friend Patricia Csaba.

I have asked Patricia to tell of her beliefs and experiences, so that I may share them here with others.

* * * * *

In the field of the Healing Arts there are therapies and modalities that are far too numerous to mention. Once a person becomes interested the door is opened and many wonderful ideas emerge.

It has always been my belief that God has given us the means and the gifts to take care of ourselves here on this earth. It is up to us to recognize and learn the skills necessary to keep ourselves spiritually, physically and morally sound. I believe we do have the innate ability to help heal ourselves.

For our spiritual health, many of us realize the importance of the Golden Rule. If we live by the words "Do unto others as you would have them do unto you" life would be a much simpler, kinder and joyful experience.

For our physical health many home remedies are simply passed down through generations and have been put to the test of time. They have been found to be tried and true.

In times past most people performed physical labor and ate more natural foods. With the onset of fast foods and modern conveniences we have morphed into a society in which we are plagued by obesity and food related illnesses.

For good physical health the basic foundations are a sensible moderate diet and daily exercise. Beyond these common sense measures I am constantly amazed at the therapies available for a healthy lifestyle.

I have worked in the Allopathic field as a Registered Nurse for some 12 to 15 years. I totally believe in good medical care, medical check-ups and sound medical advice. However I feel there is also value in the Alternative health field. I am constantly and pleasantly surprised at the therapies available for healthy living.

The fields of mainstream medicine and complementary health care could and should work together as programs integrating knowledge and skills for the good of the client.

I have been privileged to work in the Alternative health field for the past 16 years. I became interested in the mid-1990's and continue to learn and study in both fields.

In my quest for learning I have only touched upon the tip of the iceberg. I am amazed at how much and how many different modalities there are available to learn. My interest has been varied and I have studied many different types of complementary therapies. I have found most to be valid and interesting.

I do not attempt to be an expert in any one field. As I work I integrate what I have studied. So I can use one therapy exclusively or integrate others, depending on client need.

I believe that all healing comes from God. No matter what course we take we are all conduits through which any healing energies flow. We are here to serve and being in any part of the health field is absolutely a service.

Just as we change with time so does health care. I marvel at what is available through science and also what is right here in the palm of our hands.

There are so many different types of healing – spiritual, mental, emotional and physical. Keeping this in mind it is necessary to heat the whole person, not just a specific spot or illness, for one never knows where the need for healing may lie. It is in harmony that the healing happens. Harmonizing energies in and around the body allows our innate wisdom and ability to keep flowing and creates the healing balance for which we all strive.

Esther E. Hansen

Jin Shin Jyutsu is one of the therapies that I have had the pleasure of learning about and studying I am a constant student of this therapy.

Jin Shin Juytsu is an ancient art. It is the art of harmonizing the energies in the body. This therapy, this art, this Jin Shin Juytsu helps bring homeostasis to our bodies. It brings a state of equilibrium that helps promote optimal health.

This is not a manipulation of tissue and uses only light touch with the fingertips (over clothing) to assist in the natural harmony and flow of the body's energy.

I have practiced Jin Shin Juytsu as a trained practitioner and also practice self help. I have found this to be a wonderful modality for balancing the flow of the body's energies. I practice self help daily and consider myself blessed to have been led to Jin Shin Jyutsu.

I have experienced healing within myself spiritually as well as physically. I have heard of many astounding testimonies of harmonizing the life energy through Jin Shin Juytsu and have witnessed some as well. But I would like to cite one case that I personally observed and that was astonishing to me as well as an answer to many prayers.

Years ago, in May of 2008, a friend and neighbor of mine mentioned in casual conversation that her 10-year old son might be facing physical therapy and possible knee surgery to one or both knees. His diagnosis was Patella Femoral Syndrome.

He was in constant pain. He loved to play baseball and was experiencing discomfort and pain in his knees. This hindered his playing. It was especially difficult for him to run or practice the position of catcher. Besides his regular activities of daily living his ball game and play time as a boy were painful and he was slowed down considerably.

I asked his mother if she would allow me to at least try treatment before she would consider surgery. She readily consented. In lieu of payment my only condition was that he come every day for ten consecutive days.

The first couple of days she drove him over for his treatment. After that he either walked or rode his bicycle. He was asked daily how he felt and if his knees hurt. At first the knees did hurt, but gradually the pain subsided! It was amazing to me. After the 10 days his pain was almost non-existent! He was back to playing, running and baseball.

Altogether we did 16 treatments: every day for 10 days, then every other day for 4 days, then once a week for 2 weeks. After these treatments I asked him to let me know if he had any more discomfort and to come over for another treatment any time he felt he needed it, or if he experienced pain.

His mother said he was doing well and that there were no more complaints. The only thing he complained of occasionally was morning discomfort or stiffness, which also subsided with time.

There may have been many factors that contributed to the changes in this young man's condition. Prayer definitely, time maybe, but certainly Jin Shin Jyutsu helped to clear and change the energy pathways and allow the body to innately heal itself.

I love that I was given the opportunity to witness this firsthand and be an integral player in this plan. I believe that the boy also had a definite part in this because he was a willing participant in the treatments. The best part is that he did not have to undergo surgery and to this date he is well and strong and growing into a wonderfully healthy young man.

Jin Shin Jyutsu is an innate part of humanity's wisdom. I encourage you to explore it for yourself.

* * * * *

I myself have experienced one fracture. It was in no way a typical osteoporosis "break, then fall" incident. Rather, in early winter of 2007 I slipped on black ice and fell heavily on my arm, which broke.

It was wonderful to have the help of my friend Patricia to speed my recovery.

I came to her with my arm in a sling, the prescribed treatment for a fracture. Mine was a fracture of the left humerus. I was in considerable pain and was treated twice in December and regularly for a total of nine times in January before I returned to the doctor for a re-evaluation.

Patricia had determined that lymph drainage would be necessary for any swelling in and around the shoulder area. Additionally, energy balancing and energy work was used to pull pain from the affected area. Jin Shin Jyutsu was used as another modality to harmonize the body's energy. Reflexology was also incorporated in the ongoing treatment.

Her records show that I responded well to treatment, with recovery and healing well ahead of schedule. Soon the pain subsided and the fractured bone was mending well. The range of motion returned slowly to normal with minimal pain.

I went back to the doctor whom I had seen originally at the time which he had assessed to be midway in returning the arm to its normal condition. The man was amazed by the X-Rays and declared the expected physical therapy to be unnecessary.

A short time later I sent a letter to him, a copy of which is included below It tells the story of my only broken bone, and the factors that led to my happy recovery.

February 6, 2008

"Dear Dr. XXXX,

Thank you for your recent attentions. I checked with you after X-Rays in the Emergency Room confirmed that I had broken my arm on December 6. Subsequently, as prescribed, I wore the arm sling at night or when I went out. I did the arm swinging exercises three times a day. Yesterday I returned to the office for X-Rays that confirmed my own happy suspicions. You pronounced them "beautiful" and said that I was fine, with no need of physical therapy.

I must say that I was not surprised at this outcome. I am 83 years old; I have been told that I have osteoporosis, but I am thankful to have benefited from alternative healing that has kept me in good health. I walk and engage in regular physical exercise and have done this for years. Already a couple of weeks ago I felt that the arm was indeed "fine."

In the event that it might be of interest to you, allow me to list briefly the measures I have been able to take on my own behalf recently and during the past couple of years.

Since the diagnosis of osteoporosis by my chiropractor, Dr. Kerim Zouvalekov, I have been taking a dietary supplement each day containing calcium, magnesium and other minerals and vitamins. This in addition to regularly consuming another supplement from Dr. David Williams, with glucosamine sulfate and additional ingredients including herbal blends and eggshell membrane.

On consulting the Desk Reference for Essential Oils I found that there are a number of therapeutic grade essential oils whose effect is bone healing I used therapeutic grade oils of wintergreen, pine, lemongrass and vetiver on the arm each day. (Helichrysum is also strongly recommended, but it is too pricey for this senior citizen.)

I benefit from sessions with a holistic practitioner, Patricia A. Csaba, who uses JIn Shin Jyutsu and other modalities for the enhancement of bone healing, stress reduction and pain management. In January I scheduled two weekly sessions with her rather than my usual one-a-week session.

My very best wishes to you in your work.

Sincerely yours,
Esther E. Hansen"

CHAPTER TWELVE

Natural Healing Science Pioneers

Linus Pauling-- Before I knew anything at all about him, his name was associated in my thoughts with Vitamin C, a good old vitamin friend that was trusted and familiar. Seeking to know more about him led to the fascinating story of Vitamin C, a story worth telling!

Ages and ages ago people sickened and died for want of Vitamin C. Long before we had given a name to the substance that was lacking in their bodies, there was a disease that made people very sick; its symptoms were the same all over the world, and many people died of it. It was called scurvy.

The disease was known by the Egyptians 1550 years before Christ was born. We can identify it from what the ancient records tell. Hippocrates described the same symptoms in 460 B.C. And native cultures everywhere, some of them native American cultures, likewise describe what must have been scurvy and what should be given to help its victims recover.

Everywhere the same symptoms could be recognized: people became weary and depressed; they had no strength; their gums were spongy and they lost teeth, their muscles were painful; they had open wounds; the nervous system was affected. As they became worse, they developed diarrhea and fever; they had pulmonary and kidney problems. Many, or perhaps most patients died.

Who were the most likely to be affected? Sailors and passengers on long ocean voyages, soldiers on long campaigns, prisoners and those confined in workhouses or cities under siege. In more recent times, miners working in the California Gold Rush, and later

Alaskan gold miners were also affected with scurvy. Obviously, all of these people subsisted on very limited diets, with no access to fresh foods.

Sailors, whose primary foods were dried biscuits, salt pork and salt beef were the most noticeable victims. Of 160 men who sailed with Vasco da Gama in 1498 on a voyage from Lisbon, in Portugal, to India, only 60 returned. Magellan lost 208 of 230 men. Similar devastating results were common on the high seas of the world. It has been estimated that between the years 1500 and 1800 at least two million sailors died of scurvy.

There was no common substance ingested by all these differing populations. Could a common remedy be found for all of them? In the earnest, groping attempts to find one it seems as though vitamin C was discovered, forgotten, then rediscovered. It was never specifically identified as ascorbic acid--vitamin C.

While scores of sailors on the notorious Vasco da Gama voyage perished, the curative power of citrus juice was not unknown. It is mentioned in medical records of the time.

In 1536, the French explorer Jacques Cartier, whose men were dying of scurvy, appealed to the natives along the St. Lawrence River for help. He learned to save his men by giving them tea made from the boiled needles of the Eastern White Cedar tree. The needles of this tree have been shown to be rich in vitamin C.

In 1593 an admiral in the British Navy advised drinking orange and lemon juice as a means of preventing scurvy. In 1614 a handbook for apprentice surgeons on board the ships of the East India Company recommended fresh food when available, or the juice of oranges, lemons, limes and tamarinds as a substitute. The use of sulfuric acid as a last resort reflected the common conception that any acid was acceptable.

The various remedies suggested were tested in a famous experiment conducted in 1747 by James Lind of the British Royal Navy. He divided a group of 12 patients suffering from scurvy into six groups of two each. All were given the same diet, but each of the groups was provided with a different remedy. Two patients only were given two oranges and one lemon each day. After six days only these two had recovered. The other patients were still sick.

Discussion and controversy followed this first clinical trial. Citrus juice was boiled down to a syrup and given to the men of the British Navy. We know now that most of the vitamin C was destroyed in this process. Trial and error ultimately led to the selection of fresh lime juice, as the most easily available. British sailors received a daily ration of lime juice, not boiled down to a syrup, and became known as "limeys."

The British Navy was almost free of scurvy, but the disease continued to claim many victims elsewhere. Some individuals, however, paid attention and exercised common sense in protecting the men for whom they were responsible. One of these was the English explorer Captain James Cook, who ordered his men, whenever they touched shore, to gather fresh fruits, berries, vegetables and green plants. The needles of spruce trees were used to create a beverage called spruce beer. Sauerkraut was a regular feature of the menus on shipboard. Sauerkraut is a good source of vitamin C In three Pacific voyages from 1768-1780 not a single sailor on Captain Cook's ships died of scurvy.

One detour on the road to recognition of the important role played by vitamin C had come about when citrus juices were boiled down to a syrup. Another appeared when pure lime juice was exposed to air and to copper tubing. These all reduced the effectiveness of the vitamin C contained in the juice. The discovery that fresh meat also cured scurvy was likewise temporarily confusing. Instead of continued attention to the nutritional deficiency already discovered, there was a renewed focus on the search for the cause of what appeared to be an infectious disease.

Well into the 20th century the search continued on the part of conscientious scientists directed toward basic questions. Was it the presence of some negative substance that brought about diseases like scurvy, beriberi, rickets and pellagra? Or was it the absence of some positive substance that occasioned disease?

Not until 1911 were the essential substances we know as "vitamins" identified and so named. And not until 1928 was the one we call vitamin C isolated in its pure form and correctly termed "ascorbic acid."

Not until then could the simple and accurate statement be made, as it is now "Scurvy is treated with Vitamin C." The disease is extremely rare in the world today.

* * * * *

Linus Pauling doubtless traced the development of these events as related to scurvy. He will have followed too the studies and experiments aimed at exploring the effectiveness of vitamin C In treating and preventing the common cold. His own careful studies led to his book *Vitamin C and the Common Cold, which* made him the major proponent world wide, of vitamin C.

His studies revealed one of the reasons why we need to supplement vitamin C in our bodies. Dogs, cats and other animals produce their own vitamin C. Human beings don't. Linus Pauling felt that we probably did so in the past. But during the stage in human development when people ate a great deal of plant food our need for the vitamin was supplied naturally and we lost the ability to produce our own. He felt that we actually need a great deal more than is specified as the minimal daily requirement. In his nineties Linus Pauling himself was ingesting at least 18 grams of vitamin C every day.

He felt too that vitamin C plays an important role in the prevention of cardio-vascular disease and the promotion of healthy blood vessels.

I was thrilled and excited to see and hear the gentleman in person.

By the time I heard him speak in Washington, D.C. he had long-since been recognized as one of the greatest scientists of all time, and one of two - Albert Einstein was the other- of 20th century American scientists so recognized. He had written numerous scholarly works in chemistry and molecular biology. And he would become the only person ever to receive two unshared Nobel prizes, one in chemistry in 1954 and for Peace in 1962.

Linus Pauling was loved and respected as a humanitarian. He was a familiar figure among those marching in some common cause. During the Kennedy administration when he had been invited to a party in his honor at the White House, he spent the day outside carrying a placard protesting atmospheric nuclear testing. During the party that evening, he and his wife rose to their feet and danced in response to the lively music that was played. Of course everyone present was delighted.

In the presentation I heard in Washington I caught a glimpse of the real human being that Linus Pauling was. He spoke from knowledge and conviction. If he believed in vitamin C, so did I. If he advised his staff members to consume as much as they pleased of it, I would do likewise. If he was convinced that ascorbic acid (vitamin C) could prevent or minimize a cold I was ready to share that conviction.

Actually I was to experience many, many times in my life the happy effects of avoiding colds and improving my health with Vitamin C!

I learned to follow his advice and take sufficient vitamin C, and to take it at the very first minimal onset of a cold. And as to cold medicines I learned to do as he advises in his book:

KEEP THIS MEDICINE OUT OF REACH OF
EVERYBODY!
USE ASCORBIC ACID INSTEAD!

Thanks to the Linus Pauling Institute, founded by him in 1973 and now located at Oregon State University, the important research work initiated by this good man has continued. It was not only vitamin C that was recognized by him as being of major significance for human health. Other vitamins and minerals, which have been extensively explored by the staff at the institute, have been shown to help us live longer and feel better.

90 Years Young!

They have been identified as weapons against premature aging, heart disease and cancer. The prize for health research, including a monetary award. is given by the Institute in recognition of distinguished research related to preventing and treating disease through vitamins, minerals and the nutrients found in plants. It also recognizes efforts to improve public well being through spreading knowledge about health, diet and lifestyle.

A very special award was given by the Linus Pauling Institute to a man believed to be one of the greatest medical geniuses of our time.

A medical genius? - Indeed! A man who has worked quietly and courageously to combat ridicule and hostility, even a gang of thugs sent to trash his clinic. A man who has earned the respect of specialists in medical research and practicing physicians wherever his voice has been heard and his work become known. A man who has achieved international renown for his medical publications and grateful recognition from armchair readers in American homes. "Hey," they'll say. "I read an article by him in Prevention magazine." A man who also reaches out to the public on the internet. His website www.nutritionandhealing is well known; He offers health advice without charge on his "health e-tips". Those who want to know more can subscribe to his newsletter and consult his vast health archives.

This man is Jonathan V. Wright, M.D. He received the very first Linus Pauling Award for Lifetime Achievement in Natural Medicine.

Dr. Wright has an active family practice in Washington State, where preventive and nutritional medicine are emphasized. This practice is the primary focus of his attention. Tahoma Clinic combines allopathic medicine with extensive naturopathic services. The staff there includes medical doctors, naturopathic physicians, an acupuncturist, nutritionists and allergists. Many thousands of patients have been helped and healed at the Tahoma Clinic.

In addition to his medical practice, Dr. Wright has been and continues to be the author of articles and books related to natural healing and nutritional therapy. For twenty years he wrote regular columns treasured by readers in *Prevention* magazine and *Let's Live*.

With his colleague, Alan Gaby, M.D. he has developed an archive of studies in natural healing science that includes the major work published over the past 35 years. It includes nearly every major study on the subject ever published in over 350 medical journals. It would be a challenge to name some area of human health or disability that is not given attention somewhere in the archive compiled by the two men.

Related subjects. like SUGAR are also covered there. The subject attracts our attention. We may have been disquieted to hear that the average sugar consumption of American citizens is about 100 pounds per year That amounts to 20 5-pound packages of white sugar for each of us EVERY YEAR!

We note with interest some of the things that Dr. Wright has to tell us about sugar. Simply stated, there are good sugars and bad sugars. Bad sugars attract dangerous germs. One of them is the plain old white sugar we cook and bake with, and that is to be found in everybody's sugar bowl. Good sugars can disable germs. One of those is called xylitol. It is found in the fibers of many fruits and vegetables. It looks and tastes just like our regular table sugar, but it is completely different. It disables bacteria!

One place we have plenty of bacteria is in our mouths. So what did researchers in Dr. Wright's labs do? - They created a chewing gum made from Xylitol. And what happened? People who chewed the gum got 80% less tooth decay, even without changing their eating habits!

Xylitol's magic effect on the mucus membranes worked the same way on the bacteria responsible for hay fever and asthma attacks.

Researchers put Xylitol in a nose spray for people with chronic ear and sinus infections. Those miseries were slashed by 93%.

Used in other ways this wonderful sugar washed away the germs that cause urinary and bladder infections.

All of this work was with just one of the many good sugars that can be used to replace the common sweetener that we have all been over-using for years. Xylitol is not the only "good sugar". Another one is actually not technically a sugar. But it is extracted from sugar cane! The substance has been scientifically researched in Dr. Wright's laboratories and has been shown to produce welcome benefits for those struggling to control cholesterol. The sugar cane extract produces no side effects. And its cost? Just a fraction of the cost for prescription drugs.

Research is bringing about new hope for patients suffering from diabetes, heart disease, cancer. and other ills. When tested, the products of Natural Health Medicine are being demonstrated as effective and without side effects Another very important benefit is their significantly lowered cost as compared with traditional remedies.

It would not surprise us to know that researchers working with Dr. Wright love their work. It gains international attention and renown.

The use of Dr. Wright's breakthrough remedies has been taught to thousands of medical doctors, nurses and other health professionals.

Dr. Linus Pauling himself would applaud the selection of Jonathan V. Wright, M.D. as the very first recipient of the Linus Pauling award for Lifetime Achevement in Natural Medicine.

CHAPTER THIRTEEN

What Did You Say?

As people grow older, they often develop a hearing loss. Sure, you know that. It happens to other people, right? Yes, it happens to other people, and then slowly but surely, it happens to YOU!

Like many other seniors, I didn't know a thing about hearing. I remembered my father's sister from our visits in Denmark. She was a sweet, remote sort of person, who lived in a world of her own. Perhaps she was totally deaf. I don't know whether hearing help had ever been explored for her. In any case she had no hearing aids of any kind. We couldn't penetrate her world with our voices. And in her deafness she had no knowledge of how to reach out to others, certainly not to children.

Later on, also in Denmark, there was my cousin Flemming, who had been totally deaf since childhood. Like my aunt, he was always on the edge of the fun we had with the other cousins. We did not know how to communicate with him.

On subsequent visits we met him again, with his wife. They had met at the school for the deaf that they attended in Copenhagen. There they had learned sign language, could understand what we said when they studied our lips, and had also been taught to speak Though we understood the Danish language, it was hard to comprehend their spoken words. To speak your own language if you have never heard it spoken is extremely difficult. The words spoken by deaf people are not easy for others to understand. We resorted to writing, and filled endless note pad pages with our eager conversations. The affection of the young people for us was quite evident, in spite of their handicap. We knew them to be kind and loving people.

I had experienced my father's age-related hearing loss. He was given hearing aids. That was like having your vision checked and getting glasses, I assumed. Did he have any special problems? If he did he never breathed a word about it.

Now here was I, decades later, facing similar problems, and only beginning to realize that all was not quite as it should be with my hearing. A hearing loss develops slowly, and we ourselves may not perceive its existence until long after it has become obvious to others.

So my neighbors perceived my hearing loss long before I did. It was familiar territory for them. As for me, I went on cheerfully asking to have things repeated, wondering why so many people mumbled when they spoke, missing the sound of the doorbell or the telephone when they rang, turning up the TV a little louder.

One thing that bothered me was that recorded music sounded different. It wasn't quite the pleasure it used to be. There was something strange about it. Was the machine out of order? I checked this out by attending one or two local concerts. I was not eager to do that again. The music just didn't sound right.

My neighbor's hearing loss was not age-related, like mine, but it had taught her things that were important for me to know. I was thankful when she shared them.

It was reassuring to make an appointment with an audiologist who was known and trusted by my friends. I knew her to be a trained professional with an advanced degree in audiology. Her knowledge extends far beyond selling hearing aids for a franchise.

My hearing would be carefully tested in a sound-proof booth. I would be interviewed about my hearing needs and what I expected from a hearing aid. I knew that I would be offered the right hearing aid for me, from an array of reliable companies. I would expect to be able to return for adjustments or to resolve any problems I might have with my hearing aids.

There would be two of them, I learned, for our ears work together and a good audiologist sees to it that they do so effectively to give us the best possible hearing. My own idea that only one ear needed a hearing aid was incorrect.

Only those with total absence of hearing in one ear, or those with perfect hearing in one ear can justify their stance as exceptions to this general rule. Testing revealed a hearing deficit in both of my ears. I understood that two hearing aids were required to offer the best improvement that modern technology can provide.

I understood too that hearing aids do not provide the "quick fix' often achieved for vision by a prescription for eye glasses. New technology makes it possible for your audiologist, working at her computer with you and your hearing aids, to produce the best possible results for you and your hearing needs. I realized that the hearing aids worn by my father in his lifetime had little resemblance to the sophisticated instruments I was able to wear today.

Cost is a problem; these fine instruments are expensive, and neither Medicare nor most private insurance companies cover their cost. I had two friends who offered to pitch in to help me foot the bill. Hearing in my one ear is sponsored by my friend in California, the other by my friend in Holland.

Armed with some basic understanding and the necessary cash I was able to look forward to my appointment with the audiologist. She was obviously delighted to meet a new patient who was cheerful and excited about seeing her. She told me that many people struggle with feelings of denial or reluctance before they are ready to admit that they have a hearing problem and accept the necessity of dealing with it. For me those feelings did not exist. I wanted to quit struggling with the attempt to hear what was going on in the world around me ; I was happy to know that good help was available for better reconnection with the world of sound and speech.

Of course no two hearing aids are alike. Molds had to be made of my inner ears. Once they were returned to the audiologist's office and attached to the instruments they were designed to fit I would be able to return for the next important appointment to be introduced to my new hearing aids.

You have to become accustomed to the feel of the foreign objects in your ears. Do others notice the look of them? Some people are concerned about seeking out the least visible hearing aids. However, it's not the kind of thing that is of interest or concern to me.

I was much more interested in new auditory surprises. It is normal as you gradually lose your hearing to forget the world of sound in which we live With your hearing aids much of that sound world comes back to you. It isn't necessarily welcome. The fridge and the washing machine are unexpectedly loud, as are cars swooshing by when I'm out for a walk with my dog. Loud noises are unexpectedly annoying. However, I note with pleasure that I can still hear the birds; others with a hearing loss are deprived of their songs.

Glasses may resolve a person's vision problems; hearing aids, however cannot resolve all your hearing problems. I was thankful to have improved hearing, but in many ways I still had to learn to adjust in order to meet the challenges of limited hearing.

I did learn to feel comfortable about defining for others that I have a hearing loss. People are usually very willing to facilitate communication. They need to understand that it isn't necessary to talk louder in conversing with you. What does help is to have them look at you when they talk. This always makes conversation easier. I've learned to say, "It helps me to know what you're saying if we look at each other when we speak."

Trying to process very fast speech can be difficult. It may help to ask fast talkers to slow down a bit, or to insert pauses in their talk. I've learned to limit the number of guests I invite to share a meal at my house. Two couples work just fine; more than that presents a hearing challenge. Large groups are a dubious pleasure. If group discussion is planned it is never possible to hear what everyone is saying. Depending on the acoustics in the room where the meeting takes place it may even be totally impossible to hear the speaker.

Trying to hear what is perhaps a distinguished speaker in a large auditorium will very soon find me searching for the nearest exit. You hope for the best, but hearing hopes are not always fulfilled!

Restaurants present their own set of challenges for those whose hearing is limited. You ask to be seated, if possible, with your back against a wall, in a quiet corner away from the kitchen and other entrances and exits. My particular hearing aids have a setting permitting adjustment to block noise coming from behind. This can be helpful.

The internet has an increasing number of videos. They may be easy or very hard to hear depending on the tonal quality of the speaker. I am grateful for the occasional presentation with a printed version that accompanies the spoken one. Someday I hope a choice will be offered for those who are interested in the presentation: auditory, visual, or both. Like many others I can read a good bit faster than I can listen.

A few close friends may realize that listening is strenuous for the person with a hearing deficit. It makes you tired! A happy gathering of friends or family can send you home worn out from all that listening.

I learned to accept the need for an occasional rest to recover from too much auditory input!I must admit to sometimes minimizing relationships simply because of the effort that can be involved in even a brief, casual conversation.

One pleasure that I have enjoyed in all of my adult life is also closed to me now. I have always been happy to speak with children. It is sad to be forced to avoid youngsters rather than to engage in lively conversation with them. Once in a while there is an unexpected pleasure: a child whose tonal quality of voice enables me to hear what he wants to tell me!

The telephone of course demands totally attentive listening. The wonders of modern technology have not yet rendered hearing aids and telephones fully compatible. Thanks to a good friend who observed my need I have a special telephone designed for people like me. I have sometimes experienced perfect reception speaking with a friend in Holland or Ireland. Nevertheless, I may have insurmountable problems understanding what my next door neighbor is trying to tell me on the telephone. (One day I finally resolved the problem by saying, "Let's go outside where I can hear you.")

People are always willing to be helpful when you define your need on the telephone. They increase the volume, which can sometimes be effective. Or they speak more slowly--that often helps. But there are times when you have to say, "I'm sorry. I have a hearing deficit and I am not able to understand anything you are saying."

I am aware that there is a program called "Cap Tel" that permits a person to see in writing what others are transmitting with the spoken word. Why have I never investigated it thoroughly? I think because I have lived a long life attuned to the emotional qualities imbued in the human voice. I have heard the lilting joy in the voice that tells of a happy event, the shadow in the telling of grief and sorrow. These cannot be contained in the literal transmission of the written word. I want to experience those lights and shadows. I would like to hold on to them as long as I can.

Light and shadow is an inherent quality of music. I have loved music in the past, but sad to say, I am no longer able to enjoy it. I can manage to appreciate American native flute music, harp and piano music, but even these, I find, are not what I voluntarily choose for the moments when I want to listen to something.

How beautiful was the music I used to love at Christmas: Corelli, Buxtehude and Bach. And all the Christmas carols. My neighbor plays the clarinet. I love the music he brings to our Christmas Eve celebration: I love it when he accompanies my friend when she sings "O Holy Night". The first time my dog heard the clarinet playing, he ran over and sat right in front of the man who was playing. I knew just how he felt!

As mentioned previously, some people who are hearing disabled cannot hear bird song. I am glad not to be one of those. The ear, that finely tuned mechanism that captures sound waves, differs from person to person. I am glad to be able to hear the birds sing!

Another great boon to the hearing impaired is the closed captioning now almost universally available on films and television. Voices on these media are not always easy to hear and process. I appreciate those, like Brian Williams, whom I can understand without the need for captions. Women are usually less easily understood, and in many programs sound effects, changing characters, and varying voice qualities make captions a necessity for understanding. Of course, if you're reading captions you will miss other important aspects of viewing. Never mind, one learns to be grateful for any kind of successful communication!

Another hearing pleasure that I enjoy was unexpected. Earlier in life I had met with Talking Books. Personal experience with my mother, who was legally blind, introduced me to this very special service. Like most people, I had always assumed it was only for the visually handicapped, or for those with extreme physical disabilities.

Now, in my own "golden years" it never occurred to me to make use of talking books. My vision is good and I have no physical disabilities except for the hearing deficit. Hearing aids are a great blessing, but they were not able to enable me to enjoy music. At the local library I mentioned this to a librarian. "Oh," she said, "you would be eligible for talking books."

A recommendation was soon obtained from my audiologist and the application was sent to the cooperating Ohio library. It was not long before the package containing the player reached my house.

The tidy, compact machine was a revelation. Some 25 or 30 years earlier the one that my mother had was larger. It was designed for use with reel to reel tapes. The operation was not faultless, and I often had to rush to the rescue when my mother struggled with the tapes. Now I had only to insert a tape cartridge in the small, portable machine, easily regulate the volume and speed and quickly change the tape when the playing was completed.

I still have that first machine and have since added a second one--a digital player technologically designed to be ultra-simple to operate. It plays digital tapes, and a single tape contains a complete book. The machine is very small and is easily portable. There are simple adjustments for speed, volume and tonal quality. My mother would have loved these simple–to-operate tapes that can make the user fully independent.

To my great pleasure I discovered that the readers on the tapes have improved vastly over the years. Early on, dedicated volunteers did much of the reading for talking books. Now it is a real privilege to listen to readers who are skilled and experienced actors. Those like myself, for whom talking books must substitute for the music we can no longer hear, much appreciate this.

The catalogs sent to talking book users every other month through the Library Service for the Blind and Physically Handicapped contain many book choices for both the standard tape machines as well as the new digital players, which will gradually replace the other machines. Those who are visually impaired or who are physically handicapped so that holding a book is difficult or impossible can also choose magazines and. Braille books. Large print materials are also available, as well as music scores and instructional resources. All of these wonderful materials are available without charge to those who qualify for the service.

I think of my college friend, Betty, who was unable to graduate because she was bedridden with osteo-arthritis during the last year of her life. I helped her learn how to teach dyslexic children to read. The children sat beside her bed, chin in hand, eyes on the book that was positioned in a holder that both of them could see. She made a difference in their lives. Talking books could have made a significant difference in the life of the teacher and her pupils.

We can be thankful to Helen Keller for championing this wonderful service, which was established by an Act of Congress in 1931. It was available initially only for blind adults. In 1952 it was expanded to include children. Today's users comprise persons of all ages and various forms of disability.

Esther E. Hansen

I follow with keen interest the efforts of doctors exploring alternative solutions to the problems of hearing loss. Some day I hope to be able to write about a natural health product that can be of benefit to me and others who suffer with a hearing deficit.

Chapter Fourteen

What is The Healing Code?

Life has provided me with some happy experiences with what is now termed "energy healing". They have appeared, if not so categorized in these pages. Already I have described my adventures with yoga both here and abroad. It is rightly described as "creating balance in the body." Known and deeply rooted in the culture of India for thousands of years, it has provided equanimity of body and spirit to its people for many generations there. The life energy present in yoga is termed *prana*.

Now, even in small towns of present day USA it is a familiar phenomenon. As for me, I loved learning the yogic postures, though I would have been hard pressed to explain what was happening as I performed them. It was much easier to tell about how good they made you feel.

Reiki too has become popular in this country. It comes from Japan, where it was developed in modern times from ancient oriental roots. The rei portion of the name means "God's Wisdom" or "The Higher Power": the ki means "life force energy." A friend had learned the gentle laying on of hands involved in the practice. She shared her new knowledge with me so that I was able to experience the sort of radiant glow I felt in my body.

In the past, energy was recognized as crucial to all healing. It was known as the vital force of all creation. It was given specific names like *prana* and *ki*. Native American Indians had other names for it. There were hundreds of different names for life energy.

People in ancient times had sensed what was later expressed in the formula given us by Einstein in the 20th century. – everything is energy. By engaging in practices that facilitate and balance energy in the body I was learning to perceive in reality a portion of all that is meant and implied in Einstein's theory. Everything in and around us is energy--by no means least of all our thoughts.

Likewise in this astounding century the science of quantum physics was born. It is the science of things so small that you couldn't get smaller than a certain minimal amount of a thing. It is the science about which Niels Bohr, the father of the orthodox Copenhagen interpretation of quantum physics said, "Anyone who is not shocked by quantum theory has not understood it."

I have certainly not understood it. I know only that it lies at the heart of what we have termed "energy healing". It is relevant to the understanding of cellular memory. In our bodies we have trillions of cells made of energy. And these cells contain memories of anything and everything that has happened to us: recently, long ago, ever. They contain that which constitutes our likes and dislikes, our patterns of thinking and behavior, our sources of joy or stress.

According to research studies conducted by Dr. Paul Pearsall, patients who have received transplanted organs, especially hearts, frequently exhibit memories, preferences, habits and behaviors that were present in the organ donors. It would appear that these were present in the cells of the donated organs.

Are they stored only in the heart? The Bible tells us that "from the heart flow all the issues of life." We may now certainly consider that statement to be physically, not only metaphorically true. Other common expressions, long familiar, are related to this new perspective. We speak of a person with "a good heart", we do something "with all our heart". We say to someone, "Have a heart."

When such words were first spoken no one had ever heard of cellular memories; now it is not difficult to understand how the old terms are related to the new terminology.

Recent scientific studies indicate that the heart is not the only repository of cellular memories. Scientific studies deal with the human psyche. And what is that? The Greek word signifies "the vital force that evaporates at death." Most of us laymen would choose to say the soul. Experiments are conducted that deal with the psyche. They are focused on moral issues, on laughter, on hope. They demonstrate that the well-being of the body affects the psyche. A specific network in the brain is identified as dealing with issues relating to the psyche, (to the soul, or spirit) And what are these? We all know them: kindness, patience, humility, self-control and many others--the qualities that identify us as being human.

So in addition to the multiple facts we store and process in our brains, there is a part of the brain now being explored by science that is concerned with memories of what we have experienced recently or in the past. Inherent in them are the thoughts and emotions dealing with those qualities we choose to develop and cultivate in becoming good human beings. The things stored there, designated as cellular memories, are commonly identified as issues of the heart. Modern scientific research identifies the heart as being physically associated with them.

It is with these issues of the heart that *The Healing Code* is associated. The authors of this book are Alex Loyd, PhD ND and Ben Johnson, MD DO, NMD. The original impetus for the book stemmed from the information and insight provided Alex Loyd in a deeply significant personal experience on board an airliner high in the skies above the United States. This experience afforded him the answers to many desperate years of seeking the solution to his wife's clinical depression. It provided the basis for the help he has been able to offer thousands of people all over the world, similarly in search of help for healing of body or soul.

Before he obtained doctorates in naturopathic medicine and psychology, Alex Loyd was an ordained minister. He established a private practice in counseling, subsequently also in alternative therapies. For twelve years he engaged in a determined world-wide search to resolve his wife's serious health condition. His studies included exploration of quantum physics and energy healing.

Not until 2001, after 12 years of study and research, did he find what he was seeking in the discovery of a simple, physical mechanism that treats the source of stress in the human body. Following his wife's wondrous recovery, Dr. Loyd validated the mechanism through Heart Rate Variability tests. These tests are used to measure stress in the autonomic nervous system. They demonstrated remarkable success in his subjects. It was in marked contrast to results recorded with the use of other modalities.

The company called the The Healing Code was founded by Dr. Loyd to provide natural healing. The program is designed to activate the body's own stress-relieving mechanisms. It can be carried out by individuals for themselves--just people like you and me. There are no invasive procedures involved, and no diet or exercise. Dr Loyd has trained some 2000 coaches to act on the telephone to assist others in working with the procedures. Such help, however, is not essential, and many have self-conducted the program through following careful directions supplied in the book *The Healing Code*, written by Dr. Loyd along with his co-worker, Dr. Ben Johnson. A website, www.thehealingcode.com, is also available. The Heart Issues Finder that viewers can access there has been helpful to countless persons in identifying the issues most relevant to their needs in resolving their problems.

Dr. Ben Johson's name has become familiar to many through his work with the popular book, *The Secret*. He was the only medical doctor featured in the film based on the book. Dr. Johnson heard Alex Loyd speak and became interested in the work he was doing. He is a physician who describes himself as striving to offer his patients the best of both worlds. "I am combining viable conventional medical approaches with appropriate alternative therapies to create the most effective healing programs for my patients." he says. He had found that the major obstacle to wellness for his patients was dealing with the emotional, spiritual issues that remained after successfully completing standard procedures.

His encounter with Dr. Loyd led to his being able to help patients heal emotionally as well as physically. It led also to his totally unexpected recovery from a life-threatening disease. Dr. Johnson had become a victim of what we have come to know as Lou Gehrig's disease.

Even those of us like myself, who do not follow sports events, may well recognize Lou Gehrig's name. "Oh, he was that baseball player," we say. He was, indeed a renowned player with the New York Yankees back in the 20's and 30's He and Babe Ruth became headliners at that time.

Lou Gehrig developed quite different headlines when he was diagnosed with Amyotrophic Lateral Sclerosis, known as ALS, an incurable neuromuscular disease. The relentless symptoms proceed from muscle weakness, uncontrolled muscular movements, weakness of the hands and feet to eventual paralysis. Speech, swallowing and breathing are impaired, but mind and senses are not affected. After his retirement from baseball, Lou Gehrig continued to work with the parole board to help troubled youths.

On July 4, 1939, when 62,000 fans gathered for his Recognition Day in Yankee Stadium, Lou Gehrig declared himself to be "the luckiest man on the face of the earth."

Dr. Ben Johnson might well speak those words about himself. The Healing Codes healed him of his Lou Gehrig's disease. After his recovery, which involved normalization of the autonomic nervous system within minutes of time, his body was able to begin the healing process. Today he is completely healthy. He says that he knows of nothing else that addresses and heals emotional and physical issues so effectively and completely.

"It is philosophically and scientifically sound," he says. "Not to mention that it works. I'm living proof of that."

Dr. Oz, whose frequent appearances on television have earned him much popular respect, has described energy healing as being the "last big frontier in medicine." More and more people are beginning to understand the significance of energy as described by quantum physics. The Healing Codes are a quantum physics healing system that has been used successfully by individual human beings all over the world.

The system is complementary and works well in conjunction with traditional care. It does not require patients to forego medical treatment without consulting their physician. Dr. Paul Harris, who is an internationally known lecturer and alternative health expert, says of it, "This is the only area of health where there has never in history been a validated case of harm."

The book *The Healing Code* is available on Amazon, where it has attained the unusual distinction, for a health book, of being a best seller. There are over 400 positive reader reviews to be read on its Amazon site.

* * * * *

In tune with the personal nature of this book, this chapter is concluded with the personal experiences recounted by my good friend Catherine.

MY EXPERIENCE WITH ENERGY HEALING
AND THE HEALING CODES
by Catherine Smith Webner

I first heard about energy healing in the early 1990's when a friend told me she was learning the ancient Japanese art of Reiki. Reiki is an energy healing system where the practitioner seeks to access universal source energy and help it flow to the patient's body to support and facilitate the body's innate healing abilities. As my friend progressed through her training she did a few practice treatments on me. I had no health problems at that time but I was an overworked single mother of three boys who was emotionally drained after the breakup of my marriage. I was skeptical about the process of transferring energy but was open to the idea of the thought-focused healing intention of a caring person. The Reiki did not produce any dramatic results but I did feel a little lighter in mood and a little more energetic. I was already on a spiritual path for my life and had heard energy described as "the bridge between spirit and matter." The Reiki sparked a fascination in me for learning more about how everything radiates energy since everything is made of energy.

90 Years Young!

A year or so later I was told about a Johrei Fellowship Center that had opened up in my city. Another of the eastern energy healing systems, Johrei is similar to Reiki in that it is a method which enables the focusing of energy toward the body. Johrei practitioners believe Divine Light is being directed by them to the patient for spiritual purification and blessing. It intends to dispel negativity from the spiritual body and raise spiritual vibrations. Over a period of a few months I attended weekly sessions. During the first visit and every time after, while seated about two feet in front of the seated practitioner who would hold her palm up toward me, I would feel a warmth begin to slowly diffuse within my body and my nose would start to run. I was told these are not uncommon bodily reactions with energy healing. The reactions were sometimes more intense than at other times but it always felt like something was happening, I just didn't know what exactly. The practitioner said she was guided to tell me that I was storing the energy of anger in my body and that I should work on forgiveness of those who I felt had hurt me so deeply. Because of my spiritual beliefs, forgiveness was something I already knew I needed to work on but I hadn't understood how my body was being negatively affected. These experiences with energy healing were adding a higher level of awareness to my emotional life and my inner spiritual journey.

We moved away and I was busy with life when, in the late 1990's, I developed a serious life-threatening health problem. Late stage cancer. I came close to death during my nine months of chemotherapy and two months of extensive radiation, which left me damaged with permanent unpleasant side effects. I had barely survived but I was determined to do so because I had to; I had children to finish raising. While I began the slow process of recovery I searched for complementary health treatments that would assist in rebuilding my health. I was helped greatly by my friend, the author of this book, Esther Hansen, who shared her knowledge of essential botanical oils and natural health supplements. Transfer Factor played a decisive role in bringing my immune system back to working condition.

Prior to my cancer experience, I had believed that a person received traditional cancer treatment and either they died if it failed, or they were restored to good health if it was successful. Then they went on with their lives as before. I know now that there are various levels of treatment results in between those extremes. I learned that, after the physicians do what they know how to do, the rest is up to the patient to continue the healing to its best outcome.

Several years into my recovery, I came across a book called Energy Medicine by Donna Eden. This book makes clear "the fundamental law of energy medicine: Matter follows energy. When your energies are vibrant, so is your body." The book explains how to work with the subtle energies that give your body life and teaches how to do various physical and mental exercises to increase healing for yourself. I was very attracted to the idea of applying healing energy myself and to not have to be dependent upon a separate person to do it for me. The problems for me were that I had never been an exercise lover, had never developed the daily discipline necessary to do it and the chronic fatigue I was left with after cancer treatment was a deterrent. It was all I could do to take care of my children, I couldn't seem to find it within me to take care of myself too.

Then Esther found out about 'The Healing Codes'. Here was a way to apply healing energy to myself in just minutes a day that was not physically taxing! The first time I did the beginning hand movements on myself, my nose began to run slightly and I knew that healing energy had taken place. Almost immediately I felt a sense of peace and calmness and relaxation throughout my body.

I have had the Healing Codes book for about a year now and, to be quite honest, I have not explored them yet to their fullest potential. I still have days where I skip doing the codes. Some days I don't have the emotional strength to even briefly access a negative memory in order to work on it for healing. I allow the distractions of my day-by-day financial struggles to overwhelm me and then feel that working on healing is just too difficult. But I never give up.

My healing is a work in progress. A back-and-forth response is not atypical and so I try not to feel impatient or berate myself for it. I keep coming back to doing the codes because I continue to have feelings of tranquility and serenity after performing them on myself. I also see positive changes in my thinking; less worrying and more acceptance and tolerance of others. I also like the sense of empowerment I get by taking some personal responsibility for my own healing. My healing journey still has a way to go and I hold on fast to my intention to heal completely.

Our bodies and spirits are remarkable instruments of energy that have great powers for healing. We just need to persevere until we obtain our "miracles".

* * * * *****

Recent research suggests that memories and images may be stored in every cell of our bodies, like DNA. More and more people are discovering ways to access this unconscious information. Quantum Physics has brought new understandings and applications. Those like my friend Catherine who are willing to persevere will experience ever new miracles.

CHAPTER FIFTEEN

Chiropractic and Acupuncture

Friends of mine were excited about the chiropractor they had found. They had both been helped by chiropractic adjustments and urged me to schedule an appointment with their trusted doctor. "But there is nothing wrong with me," I protested. "Everyone can use a spinal adjustment at some time," they declared. "It might as well be now." They had asked me to meet them at the chiropractor's office after their treatments. There was an immediate opening in his schedule, so my decision was simplified. If there was an ulterior motive in our scheduled meeting, it was, in any case, a kind one.

I was aware that the human body is not designed to last indefinitely and that it may require special attentions with aging. I was thankful for that first adjustment and for being introduced to a chiropractor in whom I too felt trust and confidence. It was good to have recourse to his help when I experienced back problems in the years that followed that initial meeting, engineered by my caring friends. Dr. Kerim Zouvalekov (D.C.) became my first chiropractor and another valued friend.

There have doubtless been "bone setters" in many cultures throughout the world, also in ancient times, who performed various types of manipulation. The term "chiropractic" is derived from the Greek words "hand" and "practice", thus a practice carried out by the hands. Today's profession of chiropractic was initiated in this country by Daniel David Palmer in Davenport, Iowa. He was a self-taught healer who believed that the body has "innate intelligence", a natural ability to heal itself. When something interferes with the alignment of the spine it interferes with this natural ability. Manipulation of the spine can help to restore or preserve health.

Spinal adjustment manipulation is still important in chiropractic care, which also includes other treatments. There are many different types of adjustments and manual therapies using the hands or a device to apply controlled, rapid force, with the goal of increasing the range and quality of motion in the area and restoring health. Additional treatments may include electrical stimulation, relaxation techniques, rehabilitative exercise, and counseling about lifestyle factors including weight loss and diet.

Chiropractic care is considered part of complementary or alternative medicine. The 4-year program in Chiropractic training, which awards a Doctor of Chiropractic degree (D.C.), includes classroom work in the biomedical sciences and direct experience in caring for patients. Specialized training is pursued by some chiropractors in specific fields.

A local chiropractor, Alan A Newman, D.C., whom I have consulted in the absence of Dr. Zouvalekov, has graciously consented to provide some insight about his experience as a chiropractor.

My grandfather was a chiropractor in Cincinnati from the early 1930's up until 1990. I grew up there, and my whole family was given adjustments every time my grandfather came over to visit, which was quite often. I took it for granted because most of the time I was not in pain. It felt good, though. It was interesting to note, however, that I was very rarely sick while growing up. In retrospect, I have discovered studies demonstrating that adjustments can help boost the immune system significantly.

Although I thought chiropractic was interesting, I largely viewed it as something my grandfather did. However, I was interested in science and math. Engineering sounded interesting, so I pursued this and received a Bachelor of Science in mechanical engineering along with a life science minor. I was scheduled in the spring of my senior year to pursue a Masters in engineering when I came across an advertisement for a chiropractic college. I was unsure what kind of education chiropractors received, so I sent away for information. I was pleasantly surprised at what I found.

Esther E. Hansen

This sounded more interesting than pursuing engineering further at this time. With my engineering and life science background I already had most of the pre-medicine curriculum required. I looked forward to the 5 years of graduate level education, which I hoped to complete in 3 1/3 years by going year-round.

The curriculum included gross anatomy for both extremities and viscera, neuro-anatomy, neurology, clinical microbiology, hematology, pathology, pharmacology, nutrition, obstetrics/gynecology, pediatrics, geriatrics, phlebotomy, spinal adjusting and extremity adjusting among many other things. There were clinical rotations as well as a problem-based curriculum.

I remember hearing in chiropractic school about a man named Harvey Lillard who had his hearing restored by having chiropractic manipulation. The concept was that by aligning the spine correctly nerve interference could be eliminated and thus prevention or correction of a body's progression or continuance in "dis"-ease could occur. Today, most people think of chiropractic helping primarily in terms of musculo-skeletal conditions, but it can be an adjunct in helping to rectify other conditions as well, such as colic, hiatal hernia, sinus congestion and constipation to name a few.

I have felt fulfilled by my work as a chiropractor trying to help people by natural means to get better in ways alternative to drugs and surgery.

Typical musculo-skeletal problems that I have helped include: headaches--tension, migraine, cluster; sciatica; facet syndrome; sacroiliitis, neuropathy; thoracic outlet syndrome; TMJ syndrome; carpal tunnel; whiplash. Also neck, mid-back, low back, knee, ankle, wrist, elbow and shoulder sprain and strains, rotator cuff syndrome; meniscus tears; elbow tendonitis; tennis elbow; golfer's elbow, among others.

The greatest source of satisfaction in my work is seeing people get better or have a better quality of life than before. Sometimes this means an improved degree of range of motion, less pain with movement or reduced muscle spasm. A patient may walk faster, with larger steps. Some breathe more deeply or have less pain with breathing. It is good to see patients be able to prolong their careers in their chosen fields, or be enabled to play again for longer periods of time with their children or grandchildren.

I believe that each person is uniquely and wonderfully created by God. It is my job to encourage patients to attain healthier life styles and to take responsibility for the quality of their own health as much as is humanly possible. It is challenging and sometimes a source of frustration to help people understand the options available to them for alternative health care. They have to be willing to receive help and try different alternatives. Sometimes the process involved is determining what the body has as an underlying need for and then to fill it. Today people want instant results and often choose drugs to achieve this goal. Natural healing can sometimes happen very quickly, but at other times, consistency over long periods of time in appropriate healthful actions is required. Patients may need to be encouraged not to feel that whatever they attempt is not working simply because it does not work fast.

Patient experiences are individual and unique. Being used by God as a facilitator of healing is a wonderful thing. I feel that His will is always right with regard to the direction, amount and need for healing. Even the obstacles that stand in the way of healing can be opportunities for teaching and learning improved dependence and reliance upon Him in all things both physical and spiritual.

* * * * *

A sore knee was not a deterrent to a walk from my house in the village up the hill to the post office. The pain was more pronounced though, as I started home. After a few steps I realized that making it to my house was going to be a challenge. The pain was excruciating; I had to stop again and again to find a place to sit, give the knee a rest, and catch my breath. Success at last! I staggered into the house and grabbed the phone to beg the local cab company for immediate transportation.

I was thankful to see the cab arrive promptly. The kind driver helped me into the chiropractor's office. Help was certain here. The moment he was free to attend to my need "Dr Z" gave me his total attention. He identified the problem as an infection. As a friend I was able to receive the gift of a treatment with acupuncture. I was privileged to benefit from the knowledge he was not yet authorized to share with other patients. I was deeply thankful for it. The treatment was immediately effective. The pain was gone for good, and never recurred.

This was my introduction to acupuncture. The door had opened on a whole new avenue of health care--a new world I was eager to know more about. I discovered that the technique has been used in China for thousands of years. The insertion of a few very thin needles at strategic points in the body, which I had experienced in my own treatment as tiny, barely discernible pin pricks, is designed to balance the flow of energy in the body.

First viewed with skepticism in the west, the use of acupuncture has now been eagerly embraced by an increasingly large number of practitioners also in our own country. Practitioners here view the acupuncture points as places to stimulate nerves, muscles, and connective tissue. Researchers have learned that it works. It works for believers and skeptics, and also importantly, for animals. It has been shown to provide effective help for a large variety of animal as well as human ills.

The International Council of Medical Acupuncture and Related Techniques (ICMart) is an international organization comprising more than 80 medical acupuncture societies worldwide. Included are over 30,000 doctors who practice acupuncture and related techniques.

In 2005 a poll of American doctors revealed that 59% of them believed that acupuncture was at least "somewhat effective." As of 2004 nearly 50% of Americans enrolled in employer health insurance plans were covered for acupuncture treatments.

Acupuncturists must be trained and certified. Levels of training range from the master's level to an advanced doctoral degree. Certification differs in the 50 states of our country.

Dr. Newman is one of the many chiropractors who now include acupuncture as a benefit available to his patients. He speaks of this aspect of his work:

I became more intimately involved in acupuncture after being in chiropractic school in Illinois. Practicing as a chiropractor in the Chicago area I saw the added value of acupuncture. Early on I had a man referred to me who had a chronic patellar tendonitis. He had been through months of licensed physical therapy two or three times a week. Eventually he had surgery on the knee. He still had pain.

Having had only a few classes in acupuncture at that point, I was skeptical about my skills in acupuncture being able to help One treatment of acupuncture, however, and the pain never returned. My eyes got big, and I knew that there really was something to this kind of treatment.

I liked the fact that acupuncture could be used not only to affect musculo-skeletal conditions similarly to chiropractic, but also to help with systemic visceral conditions. Sometimes acupuncture is used to help with depression, addiction release, detox, digestion issues, inflammation, immune issues, among others.

Thus I feel good about this new skill. It is another way of evaluating and treating the unique and wonderful bodies that God has created. Acupuncture has provided some added avenues in order to try to help patients where other things may not have helped.

* * * * *

Patients who are aware of a need for improved nutrition may be surprised to learn that chiropractors can also be consulted for help in this area. Specific problems can result from poor eating habits or from life situations that have brought about poor health. The internet, with all its wealth of information, may be overwhelming It is normal to wonder "Where do I begin? – What should I do first?" Chiropractors like Dr. Newman can provide helpful solutions. Here's what he has to say:

Unlike chiropractic, which acts predominantly on our structural component, and acupuncture, which deals with the energetic component, nutrition addresses that part of an individual that is biochemical in nature.

All human beings' biochemistry differs to some degree. It is based on genetics, but it can also vary depending upon different stressors in our lives at any particular point in time. We may be exposed to various immune challenges, such as some form of virus, bacteria, mold/fungus or parasite. Our biochemistry can be affected by exposure to things like heavy metals (mercury, arsenic, aluminum, lead, cadmium, etc.), medications, plastic, radiation and hydrocarbons, to list a few. Sometimes the body can handle these stressors on its own, but other times it cannot, and it needs help to eliminate them. If the body's organ systems and lymphatics have been compromised due to years of improper diet, or inadequate exercise and rest/relaxation, it makes rebuilding the body more of a challenge.

Regardless of where a person may be at any given time, if he/she is still alive, there is potential for improvement. Nutrition seeks to help with this by providing the right combination of supplements in addition to teaching people to eat in such a way that it will encourage their body to heal.

How is the proper supplementation and diet determined? The body gives clues. There are many ways to plug into the body to get it to tell on itself. Blood work and urine analysis is one way, perhaps the way used most traditionally in western medicine. It has for a long time been considered the gold standard. However, when blood work and urine testing are all or mostly normal and the patient still has obvious disagreeable symptoms, other forms of testing can also provide insight.

If conditions are as yet subclinical or at least not life-threatening, traditional testing may not demonstrate abnormalities. Then, electro-dermal screening and nutrition response testing can be utilized to detect energetic imbalances. These appear on specific reflex points and/or meridian endpoints which may be affecting health. When they are balanced out nutritionally, many symptoms can be eliminated, controlled or improved. Endocardiographs can reveal how well the heart, the most important muscle of the body, is being nourished.

Other non-invasive ways of testing include heart rate variability and hair analysis, among others.

Depending on the body's specific needs as shown by testing, nutritional handling can involve whole food supplementation, synthetic vitamins or isolates, herbs, homeopathic remedies, and/or potentized water.

All programs are tested to make sure that they are in proper balance with the body's sympathetic and parasympathetic nervous system. The sympathetic part of the nervous system is the body's fight or flight mechanism. The parasympathetic part is the rest and repair portion of the nervous system. Proper functioning of both is important.

Foods that could minimize the effectiveness of the program can be tested for so that they may be avoided.

Dietary changes are sometimes made gradually. Often, people need to be retaught slowly or coached about how to eat. A person used to eating twenty Twinkies a week or 2-3 pots of coffee a day is frequently not ready to go down to zero overnight without obvious withdrawal issues.

However, people learn to "own" the changes in their diet because they begin to realize how their body feels when certain things are eaten or overdone. Often the patient becomes "in tune" with the body, and knows when it needs to be tested or rechecked.

Success in terms of potential improvement is only limited by a person's willingness to perform some degree of proper maintenance on the present vessel of his being that we call the body.

Chapter Sixteen

The Miracle of Water

What's the greatest modern invention? We are impressed by a magazine article that offers an array of recent technological wonders. What do we know about them? Are we properly thankful for what has been made available to man in today's world?

My thoughts return to the past. It is years since I first heard that very same question: "What's the greatest modern invention?" I was visiting friends on Maryland's Eastern Shore. With a quiet smile one of them asked my opinion. The answer shot back as quickly as his question:

"Running Water!" His response came with a chuckle: "Make it hot!"

The words rose up from the past in response to a water problem in my home. The usual habitual turn of the faucet in the bathroom gave no running water. The welcome gush had disappeared. Helplessly my soapy hands sought a damp washcloth. The situation was no better in the kitchen. The pile of dirty dishes looked more uninviting than ever, and more challenging!

I thought of all the daily blessings I take for granted: the flush of the toilet, the pleasure of a hot shower, the quick efficient washing and rinsing of laundry. My dog expects to find a drink of water in his dish. The plants in the windowsill are sustained by the water I give them. And I have learned that drinking water is important to preserve my own health. What now?

In the western world I need not wonder for long. A call to my plumber brings help very soon. My friendly neighbors bring me a pail of water, a bottleful to drink. They cheerfully offer their bathroom for the welcome hot shower.

Increasing numbers of fellow human beings elsewhere in the world are not so blessed. They are forced to experience the water supplies they have taken for granted slowly diminishing. I think of having to say no to a child who asks for a drink of water. I think of those who must resort to unclean water to drink because nothing else is available.

A friend who was deeply concerned about water supplies in far places went to Tanzania. His children traveled with him. For all of them it was an eye-opening experience. His teen aged son shared his father's respect for the Tanzanian people They loved life; they knew how to share with others. They were warmly receptive to those who came to help them. The distress they experienced each day about their water problems was obvious. It did not take long for the visitors from the western world to share their distress.

The lifelong respect they gained for water was reflected in the boy's comment to his mother later when he returned home. She was about to pour some unused water from a pitcher into the sink. "Mom," he said, "Don't do that! That's perfectly good water!"

* * * * *

In recent years we in the western world have learned to value not only "running water" or even "hot running water" but very simply "perfectly good water" itself. Plastic bottles filled with water have gradually appeared all around us. In a recent cartoon the kid selling lemonade takes down his sign. "Forget this," he says to his friend. "The real money is in water."

Slowly we have come to understand the value of water as something that is critically important for all of us to have if we want to stay healthy. When I was a child it was what we all drank when we were thirsty. There was plenty of it and it was free. As for its health benefits, I doubt that even my health-conscious mother ever gave any thought to that question.

We are learning that the human body actually requires lots of water.

It seems that our bodies consist of about 60 to 75 percent water. Our brains, our lungs, our muscles all need water to work well. The brain is about 90 percent water, so drinking water helps us think and concentrate better, and makes us more alert.

We must have water to regulate our body temperature. We need it to send the food values in whatever we eat to wherever they are needed in the body. Water takes oxygen to our cells. Our bodies have a lot of water, and it takes a lot of water to keep all the cells in the body functioning properly Water also helps to remove the wastes that we want to get rid of. Along with fiber, it promotes normal bowel movements.

Water helps to keep our joints and muscles lubricated, so we won't get unnecessary aches and pains. It makes us feel more energetic when we're exercising.

We need water long before we ever get thirsty. Sometimes people think they're hungry; they eat something instead of having a drink of water, which, by the way, has zero calories! It's much the better choice, by far.

We may sometimes feel sick just because we are not drinking enough water. We may feel tired or have a headache, we may be constipated, have muscle cramps or dry skin when all we need to feel better is a nice long drink of water. Personally, I've experienced poor sleep sometimes for want of adequate drinking water.

My mother's familiar motto should be extended, I think. We need to say, "You are what you eat---and drink!" And what you drink needs to be water.

* * * * *

The cartoon kid who opted for water over lemonade had it right. – "the real money is in water," and lots of folks have found that to be true. Millions of gallons of water are sold in plastic bottles all over our own country and elsewhere in the world. It sells for about 300 times the cost of tap water.

Is it any better or safer than tap water? Check out Google to verify that it's not as special as we think it is. Though some of it may be filtered or treated to some degree, much of the bottled water we buy is just tap water in a plastic bottle with a nice label. The bottle, the label, and the cost of transportation to where it's finally sold add to the cost. In a two-year study ten of the water brands tested contained 38 chemicals. They are the same ones found in common tap water.

Not mentioned in this study were the pharmaceuticals found in the water supplies of major cities, which could affect some 40 million Americans. In Philadelphia 56 pharmaceuticals were found in tap water. Studies also tend to ignore the chemicals that leach into bottled water from the plastic bottles themselves.

A little thoughtful attention devoted to these bottles and the environment reveals that 86 percent of the plastic bottles become garbage and end up in our landfills. Most of the bottles are made from petroleum products, which contribute to environmental problems and our dependence on oil. Transportation of all that bottled water contributes to air pollution and global warming.

If we need or want to carry water around. it would be a wise plan to purchase a dependable plastic bottle or metal thermos to fill with tap water. The polycarbonate bottles manufactured by Nalgene are made in the USA and have been promoted for 15 years as being safe for their intended use.

For the water that comes out of your faucet at home standards are set by the EPA (Environmental Protection Agency). If you research those standards and do not find them acceptable, you may want to explore other ways of insuring that the water you drink each day is really pure.

* * * * *

The problems associated with our drinking water must not blind us to the fact that water is a genuine gift, a true miracle for which we can and should give thanks. Of the many scientists and researchers who have devoted themselves to the study of water, I want to give special attention to two men. In their work they have told us that water is marvelous far beyond what we may have recognized as its health benefits.

The first of these men was Dr. F. Batmanghelidj. He was born in 1931 in Tehran, Iran. As soon as possible after the second World War the boy was sent by his wealthy parents to an exclusive secondary school in Scotland. He was a gifted student who went on to St Mary's Hospital Medical School at London University.

Impelled by his desire to serve mankind, he returned to his native Iran, where he at first helped in setting up hospitals and sports centers. His activities attracted the attention of the revolutionary government. He was imprisoned and had a multitude of accusations leveled against him. Eventually he was sentenced to execution.

However, it dawned on the authorities that this man could be of use as a residential doctor for the prisoners. Without medication of any kind, he had recourse to simple tap water. In his attempt to treat a patient suffering from the extreme abdominal pain associated with peptic ulcer disease, he gave the man two glasses of water. Within eight minutes the pain had disappeared completely.

The execution of Dr. Batmanghelidj was deferred. In the meantime he continued his treatment of prisoners, especially those with stress-related disease conditions. The Evin prison was "a most ideal stress laboratory" and there was no absence of tap water.

When the time for his trial arrived, he faced 32 fictitious indictments, all carrying the death penalty. As his final defense he presented to the judge the article he had written on peptic ulcer disease. The judge decided that his life should be spared so that he might continue his research.

That same article was translated and sent to Yale University, and eventually was reported on in *The New York Times*. Dr.

Batmanghelidj was released from prison, managed to escape from Iran and finally to come to the United States where he was able to report in person to scientists and researchers.

In 1992 he was invited to go to Iran, where he presented his views on television. He also addressed professionals at Tehran University and in teaching hospitals. Conditions in Iran heightened the awareness of the Iranian public to the simplicity of treating medical problems with water. The absence of drugs to treat disease also turned the attention of physicians to his ideas.

His book, *Your Body's Many Cries for Water,* was designed to be easily readable by the public. Its subtitle voiced his strong convictions: *You Are Not Sick, You Are Thirsty! Don't Treat Thirst with Medications.* This important book is still available.

It was always the hope of Dr. Batmanghelidj that the public would become aware of the necessity and benefit of water in maintaining health and addressing health problems.

Reading "Dr. B"'s book now, at an advanced age, I have begun to realize the actuality of the concepts he presents. Some of us have picked up the old formula, learned at school perhaps, that we need to drink "8 glasses of water per day." I have learned to be more specific than that. A wiser plan is to take your body weight, divide it in half and express the resulting figure in ounces. You need that number of ounces of water each day.

I weigh about 120 pounds. Half of that is 60. So my daily intake of water should be just a little less than two quarts.—When I started this program I anticipated a lot of bathroom runs. Well, that's not the case, so it must mean that my body is making use of all that water!

Do other liquids count? Does it have to be just plain water? The answer is no to the first question, and yes to the second. Liquids like tea, coffee, juices and sodas contain solvents. That means they are carrying something other than whatever is ordinarily in the water.

I picture it this way: The difference is like that between a river that has boats sailing on it and submarines below, and one that is just flowing along without any of those. For water to do its necessary work in your body it can't have extra stuff in it.

Another important concept in the book relates to our understanding of being thirsty. We think that we can tell when we need water because we experience thirst. Lots of people do; others don't. "Dr. B" tells us that being thirsty is like an emergency alarm going off at the last minute. It's the last outward sign of dehydration. If a person is dehydrated, s/he is suffering from a serious water shortage.

We know about shortages in association with serious medical emergencies. A deficiency of Vitamin C leads to scurvy; we know an iron deficiency brings about anemia. A deficiency of water leads to other serious problems. Dr. Batmanghelidj states that chronic dehydration is the root cause of most major degenerative diseases. "Etiology unknown" may mean a serious water shortage, or dehydration.

Medical practitioners, we are told, may perceive the signals sent out by the body concerning its dehydration, If chemical products are given, they can silence the signals without treating the disease condition. "Water," Dr. B's book tells us, "is the best natural medicine there is."

Clearly, it's important for us to be aware of being thirsty. Even if we're not aware of thirst, it's important to understand the need for water in maintaining our health. We require enough water, based on our weight, to avoid a water shortage in our body and to supply its needs.

Those who feel concerned about impurities or toxins in their tap water can explore the use of water filters. Yet another possibility will be presented in the pages that follow, which concern the work of Dr. Masaru Emoto, in Japan.

* * * * *

90 Years Young!

Born in Japan in 1943, Masaru Emoto graduated from the Yokohama Municipal University. He became a doctor of alternative medicine through the Open International University in India. His first book, *The Hidden Messages in Water* has been enthusiastically received. He continues to write and to lecture all over the world to listeners who are responsive to the implications of his findings.

Dr. Emoto tells of his excited interest in snowflakes. We glimpse their crystalline individuality caught on our sweaters in winter. We are told that no two of them are quite alike. They are best viewed under microscopes. Snowflakes are made of water. That would suggest that no two crystals of water are alike either.

It was his preoccupation with this thought that brought about Dr. Emoto's extensive study of water crystals. Under laboratory conditions, with results that were captured from the microscope onto film, he demonstrated the reactions of water to specific influences.

He found that water reacted in various, quite different ways, to expressions of consciousness. Water was exposed to spoken words, written words or to music. After treatment in one of these ways the water was frozen. Drops of water that had been thus treated were then viewed under normal temperatures with a microscope.

What was found was exciting and stimulating. Words like "hope" or "harmony" produced crystals that were orderly and beautiful. Aggressive words like "hate" and "anger" produced no orderly patterns. Those brought forth by exposure to classical music were beautiful. Heavy metal rock produced no crystals.

In Emoto's experiments it became increasingly evident that consciousness, expressed in spoken or written words or in music of various kinds, definitely affected the molecules in the water to which it was directed. The thoughts contained within that consciousness could be uplifting or destructive. The resulting crystals--or the absence of crystals--would tell the story.

Emoto's work went beyond the study of ice crystals under a microscope. Distance was of no importance. In one experiment polluted water from Emoto's home town became the object of the good thoughts of 200 of his students located at a considerable distance. The students were asked to direct good thoughts to the water. The water became purified by their thoughts. The intent or volition within those thoughts had a powerful effect.

Thoughts, it was demonstrated, are very real. They go beyond ourselves. They have an effect which is not limited, even by distance.

One man who was given this information responded by saying, "By showing me this you have complicated my life!"

Indeed, once we recognize the power of human thought, we are faced with the responsibility we bear as human beings. If thoughts can have a direct and observable effect on the quality of water at a distance, what about the effect of one man's thoughts upon the attitudes and deeds of others? After all, our bodies are made up of a very large percentage of water!

Can the cold, unfeeling words of a parent or teacher affect a sensitive child in such a way that it has an enduring effect on his image of himself? Can the want of sympathetic words destroy a friendship or a marriage? We need not think long before we say "of course!" in answer to these questions.

All of us can add our own experiences relative to the power of human thought and word. Youngsters who have been subjected to bullying could add their own stories here. The old saying, "Sticks and stones may break my bones, but words can never hurt me" was wrong. Words--and thoughts–can truly hurt us.

However, the beauty and wonder of Masaru Emoto's work is the demonstration of their opposite effect. Words and thoughts also have the power to heal, to comfort, to give strength and confidence.

They can encourage growth, help a person to accept his own self and the self of others. And therein lies our responsibility as human beings.

Emoto stresses the importance of our responsibility for maintaining the balance in the world around us, not only in our relationships with others, but in nature itself. Human thoughts, he contends, can create imbalance and chaos, leading to earthquakes, drought, tornadoes and hurricanes.

They can also affect what goes on here in my little house. Aware of their power, I have taped the words "Love and Gratitude" to the water bottles I keep in the kitchen. My tap water is good to drink.

Those who deride the want of "scientific method" in Emoto's work may feel it impossible to accept such ideas. For others, and I count myself among them, his work and its implications make perfect sense.

We marvel and delight at the beautiful pictures of water crystals that come from his laboratories. He urges us to choose our favorites and make them our own. Others may laugh, but we read the message in the picture we have pinned up beside the desk or in the bathroom. It can access that inner part of ourselves that we call the soul, or the spirit. It can remind us of the importance of giving and receiving that we can practice daily in our thoughts and words. It is a significant part of our wellness.

The efforts of these two men have given us valuable help for living well. Dr. Batmanghelidj has directed our attention to the need for water in the human body. He urges us to change our drinking habits. Dr. Emoto has demonstrated in unforgettable fashion the need for accepting responsibility for our human thoughts and words. He urges us to change our thoughts.

Each man, in his own way, has recognized the gift for which we can all be profoundly grateful-- the miracle of water.

Chapter Seventeen

Health Hazards in the World Around Us

My adventures in wellness have brought me benefit and blessing. After I retired from active employment there was much more yet to come!

I had not expected to make a place on my desk for a computer. It was, at first, just a handy tool. My work with a voluntary translation team was greatly facilitated by this fine instrument. The team members, widely separated geographically, were unanimously enthusiastic about being able to share, edit and perfect their work with the aid of technology. It obviated having to send countless sheets of paper on roundtrip journeys overseas.

I made the usual newbie mistakes and accepted instruction, laced by chuckles, from my more experienced, patient teammates. "Live and learn" is an increasingly relevant motto in today's world. Bit by bit, I learned, tapped reserves of patience I never knew I had, marveled increasingly at the unsuspected treasures of this new technological world. Slowly I learned to feel at home there.

Hot on the heels of my discovery of email came my exploration of the internet. I was gullible at first, ready to believe anything rendered into print before my eyes. I fell into a few clever traps before I understood that this new segment of the world was just like the rest of the world. There was good and evil here, free for the choosing, in boundless inexhaustible array. Like others before me, and still more yet to come, I made good choices and bad ones. I found much to accept and endorse, much that troubled and concerned me because I knew it to be false and evil. I began to realize that use of the internet involved making choices, and making choices involves accepting responsibility for the subsequent consequences.

Sometimes, I soon discovered, the consequences of a bad choice could ensue much more rapidly than I had previously learned to expect. And it was not always easy or possible to "ask for a refund." On the other hand, a wealth of information was available for free; I embarked on endless journeys of exploration, as one source led easily on to other associated choices. It was all a great deal easier than the encyclopedia, with its heavy tomes and countless pages of print. Here too, however, it was necessary to be aware of the need to differentiate between genuine information and unverified assertions. The discovery of "facts" that I knew to be inaccurate or untrue verified this truth for me.

In contrast to these I found the websites of authorities that I knew and trusted. They were Dr. David Williams, Dr. Julian Whitaker, Dr. Jonathan V. Wright and others. The newsletters they offered were dependable and informative. I soon found "on the web" the companies I knew to be trustworthy: Young Living with its essential oils, 4LifeResearch with its Transfer Factor. In time, I learned the ins and outs of creating a website to promote the fine products in which I believed.

Those who can afford to own a computer, or make use of it at a public library, are free to enjoy its advantages. E-mail is a cost-free and efficient means of rapid communication. It became one more valuable tool in the translation work I was doing. Use of the internet is not compulsory, but for me it became an extremely important source of knowledge and information.

* * * * *

I was especially attentive to information about cancer. A beloved niece had succumbed to the disease before either of us was aware of anything other than what was offered by allopathic medicine. Another relative, who became a close friend, had opted out of the traditional radiation and chemotherapy. When I became involved in helping her find the right alternative help we were given wise counsel and she became cancer free. Now another friend was actively involved in seeking and applying alternative help for leukemia.

My internet explorations led me to an organization called *Cancer Defeated*. It is a private, for-profit publishing endeavor, founded in 2006. What it does is to research, investigate and report on alternative cancer treatments. Recently it has promoted a book by Tanya Harter Pierce, M.A., MFCC called *Outsmart Your Cancer*.

Have you experienced the intuitive perception that tells you without a doubt that something is RIGHT, and what to do about it? It was the feeling I had at once when I saw the name of this book. I wasted no time in ordering it and having it sent to my friend. I told her about the book and that it would be coming as a gift to her. "Well...thank you, but I already have so much information..." Those were her first words, but since then I have been thanked at least a dozen times for the book *Outsmart Your Cancer*. She is following a treatment option offered there, and has purchased additional copies of the book to give to others.

The author of *Outsmart Your Cancer* has a lucid, uncomplicated way of sharing the knowledge she has assimilated and made her own. In dealing specifically with cancer "triggers" she shares facts that all of us can use in understanding the health hazards that confront us in today's world, whether or not we are battling cancer. The comprehensive insights she provides have been helpful to me in defining for these pages some of those major hazards.

Here in the United States we regularly encounter health dangers related to food. The very food we eat can be a hazard. We must be alert and aware in order to escape everyday hazards in today's world.

Most of us tend to be in a hurry. We don't want to spend a lot of time with food preparation. Grocery stores are loaded with processed foods that cater to our preferences. Lots of quick and easy to prepare foods come in a box. Any food that comes in a box is also liable to be significantly short of vitamins, minerals, fiber and other nutrients.

Many of us fail to eat enough fruits and vegetables. And when we do, the plants that produced them may have been grown on depleted or contaminated soil. Depleted soils are those that don't have the proper balance of minerals in the chemical fertilizers used. Herbicides and pesticides are added to the soil or sprayed on to the good things we like to eat. They go into the fruits and vegetables. They can't be washed off. That is one good reason why those who can afford it choose to purchase organic foods.

It is sad to contemplate the fact that there is no soil on earth that is immune to the negative effects of human activity. Where is there any pure, uncontaminated soil? It is to be found, I read somewhere recently, only in the almost inaccessible depths of the Amazon Jungle. Even organic farmers cannot escape the sad reality that no soil is 100 percent pure.

* * * * *

Another food hazard that is relatively unknown is termed GMO food. What is that? The letters GMO stand for "Genetically Modified Organisms." Genetic engineering means taking genes from one species and inserting them in another. For instance, it would mean taking genes from a fish that does not freeze in icy waters and putting those genes into a tomato plant to keep it from freezing.

Foods produced from the genetic engineering of seeds are the result of experimentation. The seeds have not been tested for their effect on human beings. Independent testing of these products is not required by the FDA.

GMO crops kill beneficial, necessary insects. GMO crops cause sterility in the soil. GMO seeds have pesticide inside them. It cannot be washed off. Farmers who use GMO seeds must pledge not to save seeds. Seeds must be repurchased from Monsanto, the corporation that distributes them. In cases of crop failure, small farmers have been known to commit suicide as the only solution to the disaster.

Most other countries have banned the use of GMO seed products and foods. In most industrialized countries genetically engineered foods must be labeled as GMO. In the United States this is not the case. GMO ingredients are now in two thirds of our food. Deaths and near deaths have already resulted from GMO foods. When they were polled, nine out of ten Americans said they want GMO labeling.

The facts in the above statements have been culled from the carefully researched book by Jeannette Russell, *How to Survive (and Thrive) in a Toxic World*. After the death of her thirteen-year-old daughter from bone cancer she was motivated to give expression to what she was able to learn about the contributing factors to her child's fatal illness. Her book is a conscientious rendering of facts that also includes specific information about what you and I, as concerned Americans, can do with the knowledge.

* * * * *

We do assimilate certain generalizations from TV and other sources. We have learned to avoid high fructose corn syrup. Many are aware that refined white sugar is bad news for the human body. Recently I heard a young woman proudly assert that she had given up sugar altogether. Ready to congratulate her, I was shocked into silence by her next statement: "And I drink diet-cokes!" Like sugar, diet sodas are bad news for the human body. They contain artificial sweeteners like aspartame, also known as Nutrasweet, Equal and Spoonful.

Studies have shown a very clear connection between aspartame and various kinds of cancer, especially brain cancer. Yet millions of people in the U.S. consume products containing aspartame every year. There are over 5000 products, not only sodas, that contain it. Some of us are learning to read labels and watch for this sweet poison! This is especially important for parents to watch in purchasing syrups, antibiotics and vitamins for children. These frequently contain aspartame as a sweetener.

* * * * *

We can become label-readers, perusing the small print that identifies the ingredients in the item we contemplate buying. We can easily drop diet cokes and other drinks that may contain toxic sugar substitutes. But we cannot drop water! It is perhaps our beverage of choice. Or do we prefer juices, beer or wine? They may have been made from water that was fluoridated. <u>Fluoridation</u> is another significant health hazard, especially so in the United States.

In the book *Outsmart Your Cancer,* the author tells in detail the extraordinary story of fluoridation. In brief, science had provided the information that one type of fluoride could prevent tooth decay. It was determined that fluoride would be added to our water supplies. It also began to appear in common dental products. However, the type of fluoride added to our water supplies and toothpaste was not the same type used in the previous scientific experiments. It was, instead, a type that is a proven carcinogen.

This toxic substance is now in the water coming out of water taps in many places throughout the U.S. It may be in the water people drink, in which they shower and bathe their babies. It may be in the fruits and vegetables they eat, the flour used in baking. It may be in many other beverages and, of course, in tooth paste.

In checking the colorful array of dentifrices offered by the local supermarket I was able to find NONE that were without fluoride. At the health food store I discovered a product without fluoride that contains xylitol, a beneficial sugar substitute derived from plants.

Most European countries do not have the water problem. There, only 2 percent of the people drink fluoridated water. It has been banned or rejected in one country after another since 1971.

* * * * *

Another health hazard discussed in *Outsmart Your Cancer* is one that most of us have hardly been aware of. It comes to mind, though, when water is mentioned. In many places in our country, people are very much aware of the disagreeable taste of chlorine in drinking water. It is used to disinfect the water so people won't succumb to the microbes that cause diseases like cholera and typhoid fever. For the same reason, chlorine is used in swimming pools.

In the past, carefully controlled laboratory experiments had demonstrated that chlorine was quite safe. It did not produce cancer in laboratory animals. It broke down harmlessly into salt and water.

But in the 1970's scientists made an alarming discovery. There were toxic chlorine by-products in drinking water formerly considered to be quite safe. Where did they come from? What was happening was that the chlorine in the water combined with organic materials, especially where the water sources were reservoirs, lakes, and streams. The products of that combination were called organochlorines. Once produced, these are very stable, last a long time and are easily absorbed by animals and human beings. After a while they accumulate in fat cells and cause birth defects, immune system breakdowns and cancer.

Filters have been set up to remove organic materials before chlorine is added to public water supplies. Shall we breathe a sigh of relief?

Perhaps, if your crystal clear water comes from a nice well on your own property. But organochlorines can also enter through your skin in the swimming pools you frequent. You can breathe them in through the steam emitted by your dishwasher or washing machine, and quite possibly, simply by eating certain common foods.

One of the most powerful of the organochlorines is a group called dioxin. This category is identified as the most carcinogenic type of manmade chemical known to science. One source of dioxin results as a waste product of the paper industry. Dumped into streams and waterways it is absorbed by fish and by food crops consumed by animals. We absorb this dietary dioxin from the meat, fish and dairy products purchased at our supermarkets.

Again, Europe is well ahead of us in dealing with this large problem. There, other procedures are used to displace chlorination of drinking water and other public water supplies.

90 Years Young!

* * * * *

Health hazards that invade the air we breathe are also discussed in *Outsmart Your Cancer*. They are beyond the scope of individual action, but it is important to know that they exist. We may have the opportunity to participate in organized group action to counteract them, based on scientific fact.

One of these hazards is asbestos. – What? Didn't we solve that problem a long time ago? - Yes, to some extent, but the problem has not gone away. There are still thousands of buildings, all the way from skyscrapers in New York City (2/3 of them are included!) to schools throughout our nation that are insulated with asbestos. Its miniscule fibers are still breathed in by men, women and children everywhere in industrialized countries. U.S. government officials have estimated that 10 to 15 percent of all cancers are caused by asbestos.

The use of asbestos has been replaced by fiberglass, which is believed to be just as cancer-causing. 90 percent of all the homes in America are insulated with fiberglass.

One additional hazard is still with us, though we would prefer to forget that it exists. Nuclear fallout from tests conducted in Nevada caused cancer in many persons living or working there in the 1950's and 60's. Radioactive nuclear fallout has been windblown across the globe from nuclear testing or nuclear disasters elsewhere in the world. These radioactive substances in our air, our soil and our water will continue to affect life on earth for a very long time. The health of thousands of people has been and will be negatively affected by radioactive compounds.

* * * * *

Fortunately, there are those health hazards in modern life over which we do have some control. It has not been my primary intent to speak of health hazards, but rather of the pleasures of physical health. Over time it has become more important for us to be aware of the hazards if we wish to enjoy the benefits of wellness.

Those who are smokers today must surely all realize that they engage in a hazardous habit. 30 percent of all cancers in our country --not just lung cancers, but many other cancers that are linked to the habit, are attributed to smoking, actual or passive. The Greek doctor I met years ago identified the effect of smoking by pregnant women on the children who subsequently become learning disabled.

People are becoming more aware of our national addiction to sugar. They are beginning to recognize that there are good sugars and bad, and which are which. Xylitol and stevia are words that have been welcomed in our vocabularies. We look for honey and are also pleased to find Grade B, the best of maple sugars, at the health food store.

And while we are there we check out natural health support for sinus protection and pain relief. We discover xylitol toothpaste and nasal spray. We find seeds and nuts to substitute for the processed crackers that have been our habitual health-threatening snacks.

Perhaps we decide to try out White Willow Bark or Devil's Claw as pain relievers. We ask about valerian and melatonin products to induce natural sleep.

At the grocery store, if we can afford it, we seek out organic foods.

We learn to avoid processed foods. We check labels carefully for words we hope to see, or for others that cause us to put the item back on the shelf.

We dare to examine frankly the personal health habits that may have interfered with the joy of healthy living - the personal everyday habits that may have become health hazards. We may venture an honest look at the issues of the heart that are basic to the stress that causes many health problems.

There are books already mentioned in these *Adventures in Wellness,* that can be helpful in defining and dealing with health hazards. They can be found, along with others, in the Bibliography at the end of this book. The newsletters distributed by the trusted doctors, Williams, Whitaker, and Wright also extend invaluable help to readers dealing with health hazards.

The website I established together with my friend, Catherine, is called www.theshiningswan.com. There important health resources can be found through the companies Young Living, whose primary products are life-giving therapeutic grade essential oils and 4LifeResearh, whose flagship product, Transfer Factor, is essential for maximal immune support.

On the internet we may add our voices to join with others in protest or concern regarding current health issues. Such opportunities are provided and comprehensive information is given on Citizens for Health and Natural Solutions Foundation.

We learn to value health practitioners like those who practice reflexology, Jin Shin Jyutsu and other holistic therapies. We recognize the help they can provide when we have been assaulted by life's health hazards. And those, like myself, who are in the "golden years" may especially value the support they give to maintaining physical health and avoiding its hazards.

We learn to seek out, as well, the support of medical professionals, whether traditional M.D.'s, homeopathic physicians. or others who afford complementary or alternative help. We learn to trust them. We learn to listen to our own bodies so that we can work constructively in cooperation with those from whom we seek advice.

Each and all of us have our own stories to tell – our own adventures in wellness.

CHAPTER EIGHTEEN

Staying Healthy Through the Years

I write these words on the screened front porch of my house. There are flowers around me, growing in pots and hanging baskets. It is my favorite place for breakfast during the summer months. Insects cannot interfere with the enjoyment of the meal I have before me here. I glimpse the flutter of birds, the occasional passage of a butterfly or humming bird among the roses of Sharon that are in full bloom just now.

The porch garden is ideal for seniors like myself. Caring for growing things is a happy occupation, and there is just enough of it to be a joy and not a burden. There is an occasional scampering squirrel or a wren nest-building in the impatiens that fills the flower boxes at my windows. Recently I watched a doe with two fawns on one of those little tours that the deer sometimes conduct through the village. Here in my little porch world I can be in touch with nature, without having to suffer the assaults of sun, wind, and weather cheerfully endured by the younger generation.

This day, however, it was tempting to go farther afield. There is no better time for a walk than in the gratifying cool of the early morning. Others felt as I did. I hailed a senior couple I know; we exchanged congratulations on having chosen to walk at this early hour.

As long as I had a dog there was, of course, no need to ponder the choice. A dog tells you quite clearly when it's time to GO. There was no need to wonder whether we should take a walk. We set forth in the best and worst of weathers, and both of us felt better for doing so.

Returning from my walk, I wanted to add my usual physical exercises to the morning's agenda. They require only ten or twelve minutes of time, and inevitably leave me feeling thankful for having made the effort. First the Edgar Cayce Head and Neck Exercises, then the five "Tibetans" in my customary abbreviated version. After completing them I feel energized and well prepared for the demands of the day.

Morning seems to me the best time for exercise, though walking can take place at any time during the day, sometimes depending on the weather. Being without a car takes me to the post office on "the disciples' horses" no matter when I go. And that's a good thing.

Exercise, in one form or another, has always been part of my life.

There's something for everyone. One of my senior friends opts for her bed as the best place for the arm and leg exercises that are right for her. Others choose to take advantage of the machines available at the nearby college health facility Swimming is another favorite choice.

Whatever you do it seems to me very important to do it regularly. Your chosen exercise needs to happen every day, every other day, three times a week...whatever!

Of course you go walking if you have a dog. But dogs make other contributions to our well-being. My many years as a dog owner have taught me that. When you find the right dog for you, you gain a loyal friend. He or she will love you and trust you. They know you can be depended upon to care for all their needs. You'll know that every dog is different. You'll do whatever this one wants and needs. The two of you will be connected. And that's important! Being connected with a dog makes you feel good. It teaches you to be caring...to be a better human being.

Of all the dogs that have come to live with me there was only one with whom I didn't hit it off. I felt guilty, as though it was somehow my fault Finally, though, I had to give it up. I called the lady, the rescuer from whom I had procured the dog. She reassured me at once. "Don't feel guilty," she said. "This dog will be the perfect one for somebody else."

Cats are good pets too, though they are usually less personally associated with you than dogs. But they fulfill an important need, part of what supports your good health. I think it is important for us to be somehow in touch with nature. It is a need experienced in one form or another by all human beings. For me, it is easy to fulfill the need on my front porch, or with walks on the quiet village streets or the nearby nature trail. During the years when I lived in big cities it required potted plants in the window sill, or visits to the park.

It is interesting to know that Central Park, in New York City, was begun with that very need in mind: to be in touch with nature, to relax and to meditate. In 1857 it was a huge tract of land, far from civilization, between New York City and the village of Harlem. It was destined to become a park like those in Paris and London. The design chosen as the winner of a competition had large meadows and hills, with lakes and bridges, pedestrian walks and roads. An enormous number of trees was planted. It took 20,000 workers 15 years to complete the project. In time, playgrounds and sport facilities were added, as well as tennis courts, baseball fields and theatres. The Central Park Zoo and the Metropolitan Museum of Art were incorporated.

Central Park experienced a period of decline associated with physical danger to those seeking rest and relaxation there. Since that time it has been renovated and is once again pretty much a clean, safe place for the people of New York City.

Another major effort in our country has been the "rails to trails" project that has created safe, scenic trails for pedestrians and bicyclers in the places formerly occupied by rail lines. I love my walks on the trail near my house, with or without a dog. Trees unite in green arches overhead, wildflowers blossom along the edges of the trail. There are families out for Sunday walks or bicycle rides, moms and dads with baby buggies, young lovers, and happy seniors. There are lots of smiles. On foot or on wheels people using the trail feel good!

90 Years Young!

* * * * *

Beekeping is hardly an expected avenue, in the big city, for being in touch with nature. I was fascinated recently by an article in our local small-town newspaper on that very subject. It discussed the recent growth of beekeeping as a hobby, especially among young people.

An illustration showed two beehives in a rooftop garden planted with wildflowers and native grasses. They are located atop an eleven-story building in Chicago. Apparently hives can be found everywhere in Chicago wherever flowers are at hand. And people are planting flowers and organic gardens, free of pesticides. Is there any honey? Absolutely! Already this year, it seems, one of the hives has produced 200 pounds of honey over and above what will be kept to sustain the bees through the bitter winter.

I am not inspired to keep bees, but it is exciting to contemplate the rebirth of this ancient skill as a new and useful hobby, that surely puts its practitioners in touch with the world of nature. Quietly I contemplate my modest porch garden, and think of its contribution to my own health and well being.

* * * * *

In addition to contact with nature I have mentioned the importance of pets and regular exercise in keeping a person healthy. Another important factor in supporting and maintaining my health has been good, natural sleep. I have been blessed, all my life, with the willing acceptance of "lights out" at an early hour College reading and assignments were completed just as readily by "dawn's early light" as in the all-enveloping darkness after midnight. I was happy to keep "Cinderella hours" well before others were ready to leave a party. A shipboard romance was confined to the daylight hours. My erstwhile partner, who had cherished other plans for the night, voiced his surprise, "You really do fold up when it gets dark, don't you!"

I'm happy to be numbered among the larks, the "early to bed, early to rise" crowd. We rarely see a great many stars, but we have many a lovely sunrise in our store of memories! Whether you're a lark or a night owl, sleep is something you need. Anything you can do to encourage gaining and keeping it is important. I was struck recently by the statement I read that good, regular sleep is related to maintaining a healthy immune system. Those who sleep well think more clearly. They are better able to meet the day's demands with energy and patience.

Even larks can experience problems with falling asleep from time to time. My experience at such moments has persuaded me that keeping a regular schedule of slowing down at the end of the day is worthwhile. Let world events pursue their varied courses without your participation. Turn off the TV and anything else that may be stimulating. Close down the computer. Play soft music Call to mind from your days of "English lit" the lines of Wordsworth:

> "The world is too much with us: late and soon,
> Getting and spending we lay waste our powers:
> Little we see in Nature that is ours......."

We all have our own ways of closing the door on the world and all its "getting and spending". Each of us can find his own. When the evening is cool enough I'll go onto the front porch and sit quietly in the oncoming darkness. Sometimes a cup of tea can help to promote the necessary relaxation. Chamomile tea is good. Or a cup of warm milk with honey. Products borrowed from nature can be helpful: melatonin and valerian are old, trusted remedies, to be found at the health food store. They are components of a sleep-inducing product offered by Dr. Julian Whitaker. It is called Restful Night Essentials.

Jonathan V. Wright has good advice involving tryptophan for those whose insomnia is linked with depression.

Some people choose pharmaceutical remedies. It would not be my choice if I had serious problems with sleeping. I would seek advice from a naturopathic or Homeopathic physician. A good night's sleep-- every night--- is very important. It's worth the effort involved to make sure we get it.

90 Years Young!

* * * * *

I've experienced all the usual feelings about food. I love it when someone else does the cooking; it's no fun at all preparing a meal for myself alone. Life has taught me all kinds of useful things about nutrition. I know which foods I should eat to stay healthy, and I don't always follow the rules that life has offered me.

For those who need to learn the rules, the computer makes it easy. You access the website www.choosemyplate.gov. The plate they want you to choose on this site, sponsored by the U.S. Department of Agriculture, is the new icon recently unveiled to take the place of MyPyramid. It's a simplified version of the nutrition program formerly displayed there. The plate is divided into four sections and labeled fruit, vegetables, grains and protein. Click on any one of them and you will be transported to an impressive array of information designed to answer any question you could possibly come up with regarding that subject, from simple definitions to recipes featuring the food group selected.

Uncle Sam is clearly outdoing himself in trying to keep the public informed, and if we fail to follow his wise advice it's no fault of his!

Our food choices, though, are a matter of habit, and given the present state of our economy, they are also often a matter of how much money we have to spend on food. Choosing wisely requires thoughtful judgment, based on what we may know is <u>right</u> to choose, along with what we are <u>able</u> to choose.

For those who are interested and willing, it can be very purposeful to explore the acidity and alkalinity of our own bodies and that of the foods we select as major or minor portions of our diet. There are excellent books available on the subject. They offer the results of research in this area and suggest specific steps to take in dealing with nutrition from this aspect. Book titles are available in the appendix of this volume. This kind of approach can be especially helpful to those suffering from conditions that respond especially well to nutrition, geared to support and ameliorate health problems.

For some it can be interesting and beneficial to explore the ins and outs of eating right for your blood type. There is a helpful series of books---one for each blood type----with specific information about which foods are right for each. You might want to try a series of meals with a friend with whom you share the same blood type. I did this once for a few weeks, preparing the meals that the two of us shared. It's a good way to get started, if this is your inclination.

For the rest of us, these general rules can apply: Avoid the obvious food hazards, like sugar and refined white flour. Stay away from processed foods insofar as possible. Try to maintain a sensible, well-balanced diet, with not too much or too little of anything, Take an honest look at your food habits. Deal with them one at a time, systematically replacing bad habits with healthier ones. Eat as well as may be possible for you. We can all do something to improve the way we eat if we decide to make the effort.

If you decide to go for professional assistance, the person to seek out for dependable advice is a nutritionist. Remember the woman whose advice about nutrition was so important to my mother in the 1930's and 40's? A nutritionist is like a modern Adelle Davis.

* * * * *

My preference here is to deal not with its content but with the meal itself as a health-giving entity. I have experienced it in that way myself, as an opportunity that can contribute in a meaningful way to our health.

I recall the agreeable meal times of my childhood and youth – the times when we gathered together as a family. Sometimes there were events of the day to be shared; sometimes there was nothing in particular. But we were united in the homely, familiar rituals associated with sharing the good fare prepared by my mother. It was never a hurried meal.

Good manners were part of the ritual. We all read books, magazines, newspapers, but never at the table. If there was demanding school work to be done, you asked politely for permission to leave the table Mom had prepared the meal ; it was normal for children to take care of the dishes.

Breakfast was less leisurely, but simple formalities were observed.

Nobody stood up to eat, or dashed off with coffee cup in hand.

Surely our meal times played a part in the development of a normal, healthy digestive system.

Christmas Eve dinner was memorable. The food was unforgettable.

But it was the reverence that pervaded the meal, with like-minded people experiencing it together, that was an integral part of it, that made it like none other in all the year.

Birthday celebrations were rendered more festive for being supported by the dependable structure of everyday life, and the birthday person was made to feel especially important. You knew yourself to be very special, surrounded by the loving attention of those who cared about you.

I recall the many times in my life when the sharing of a meal was a time of shared emotion – companionship or grief, joy or sorrow. One childhood memory remains especially clear. The year was 1937. I was with my mother and sister in Denmark----the last of my childhood visits there before the German occupation in 1940. Dark clouds were gathering over Europe. I had been unaware of them; I was still a child, with none of the maturity that others might achieve by the age of 13. A number of family members were gathered around a large table for a meal. There was not the usual laughter and joking. There was a sense of heaviness in the air. I felt it and saw that some of my aunts were crying. I could not grasp the why, nor understand the unusual emotion of which I became a part. The occupation was still three years away, but the handwriting was on the wall. Only later did I remember the scene of that shared meal. I knew that having the meal together was something that cemented the family bond.

There have been other meals in which emotion played a part – not always with family. I recall the bonds established among students in Switzerland around a steaming pot of fondue. The normal Swiss reserve vanished as the chief cooks melted cheese, added Kirsch, and cut the crusty dips of bread ready to be swirled in the hot mixture.

It was the first time I experienced the bond of friendship with the Swiss students who had not previously been my friends.

It was in Switzerland too that a similar bond was established with a young woman whom I had not known fully until that day. We were high in the Alps, in a restaurant established with a full view of the adjacent glacier. It filled the windows before us as we entered, offering the first full view of it that I had had. I was totally overcome, speechless with wonder. The waiter came to ask if we were ready to order. "Not yet," said my new friend. "She has never seen a glacier before." The depth of friendship was cemented by her words. The man nodded and withdrew quietly until later. We had a very special meal together.

I shared another special meal with friends in Holland. I sat with the couple in their beautiful home, where the view from the windows was of the beautiful Rhine, with all of its varied river traffic. The simple joy of being together was with us all. He turned a smiling gaze upon me and said to his wife, "Our Esther...." The two of them and our sharing of a meal together are a beautiful memory.

After a funeral, here in the United States, the family often gathers to share a meal made of the food donations given by friends. We had experienced my mother's funeral, and received the many friendly words and condolences of so many who joined us there. Now we sat in the evening around the table where we had so often gathered for festive meals. The meal was good, and there was no work associated with it. We were basically quiet, sharing a few impressions of the day.

My young nephew turned to me: "This is wonderful," he said. It was.

A meal can be much more than simply food. Food can be downed in a hurry at a counter or handed out through a window at a fast food place to passengers who are in a hurry. It does not require fancy food and festive surroundings. It can be a gathering place for human hearts in love, affection or friendship. It can nourish and sustain human health. I am thankful for all the times I have experienced that in my long life!

* * * * *

Here on planet Earth we are surrounded by physical dangers. No one of us is invulnerable to them. We can succumb at any moment to the threat of disease and disaster. How can we defend ourselves?

Those who have survived physical assault – the power of evil in pain and torture, starvation and deprivation, speak of the power of human giving and receiving. Those who have suffered sudden unexpected disaster also understand that power. The scientists speak of the power of affirmative emotions. We can experience them at special or unusual times and each day in the simple rituals of living. Giving room to "affirmative emotions" – even at meals, contributes to our health. I have experienced this to be true.

CHAPTER NINETEEN

Tomorrow's Physician

In January 2009 a group of distinguished professionals collaborated on an article that appeared in the New York Times. At that time the headline of the article was attention-getting: "Alternative Medicine is Mainstream."

Joining forces with Deepak Chopra and Andrew Weil, whose names are familiar to many, were Dean Ornish, clinical professor of medicine at the University of California and Rustun Roy, a professor emeritus of materials science at Pennsylvania State University. All of these men were known and respected in the medical world. Their books are read by those of us "just folks" who are curious or eager for information about health.

In their article the authors emphasized the importance of moving beyond the debate of alternative versus traditional medicine. What is important, they said, is to focus on what works. This has nothing to do with the affiliations that divide human beings, like politics. It is focused on issues common to us all. It is related to medically effective treatments that have also been proven to be cost effective.

Included in what is called "integrative medicine" they said, are the best of conventional approaches, as well as alternative therapies like yoga, acupuncture and herbal remedies. They cited the health convictions formulated by then president-elect Barack Obama and former senator Tom Daschle regarding the need to address the fundamental causes of health and illness. Their health plan urged the provision of incentives for healthy ways of living rather than reimbursing only drugs and surgery.

The authors of the *New York Times* article emphasized that simple choices about what we eat, how we respond to stress, whether or not we smoke cigarettes, how much exercise we get, along with the nature of our relationships and the social support we have can be as important as drugs and surgery.

They cited studies demonstrating the enormous cost of treating chronic diseases that had already occurred. Such diseases might well have been prevented, or even reversed, they indicated, by health care rather than disease care. A study reported in September 2004 in *The Lancet* followed 30,000 men and women on six continents. It found that changing life style could prevent 90 percent of all heart disease.

The authors cited the obvious benefits to be derived from choosing a healthy life style. It can make us live longer and also live better. Experience in my own life has verified the truth of what they say. I have learned for myself <u>what</u> <u>works</u>. Some bad choices have helped me to make better ones. In reading and in real life I have met people worthy of respect in the field of health.

I understand the important role of personal responsibility in living well.

It is an essential component of working successfully with those who help us to be healthy. I recognize too that health professionals of diverse kinds will increasingly work together to serve the needs of human beings.

We are living at the dawn of "Integrative Medicine". What does that mean? What can or should we expect of those who are physicians in the world of tomorrow? I have asked a few people to voice their thoughts and opinions about "tomorrow's physician" in print. I value their words in addition to what has already been stated here.

* * * * *

My niece, Catherine, shared her experience with The Healing Codes in the chapter bearing that title in this book. She held a responsible position in one of the many offices of a large, well-equipped hospital in Arizona. She became a patient in that same hospital, where she was provided the orthodox radiation and chemotherapy treatments for lymphoma. Now, years later, she wrote to me as follows:

'Tomorrow's physician' will be the most advanced healthcare professional in modern history. The future doctor will have, at fingertip access, extraordinary and instantaneous computerized diagnostic capabilities.

Surgeons will continue to perfect exacting, targeted operations with newer lasers and robotics while being minimally invasive to our human bodies.

Researchers will have honed their skills in stem cell therapies, with their many promising applications. We will be able to replace our diseased or injured organs with replacement organs formed from our own stem cells, making the current use of transplanting organs from others' bodies obsolete.

New antibiotics and other safe medications and supplements to combat commonplace diseases of today will have been created.

Gene therapy and DNA manipulation to eradicate birth defects and inherited disorders will be used judiciously and ethically in eradicating birth defects and inherited disorders. New understandings related to careful study of mineral and nutritional deficiencies will be the primary method of bringing young and old alike to optimum good health both physically and emotionally.

Medical colleges will be graduating physicians with intricate knowledge of the interaction of nutrition and health. An integral portion of the open-minded education they receive will be the knowledge of alternative and traditional methods and treatments.

All this wonderful technology will not, however, provide us with an ideal future physician unless we retain some of the healing wisdom of the past. Total healing cannot occur in a vacuum of science. It is an intertwining of body, mind, and spirit. There is no substitute for simple human touch and the healing validation felt by a patient who is being listened to with compassion. Doctors must be provided with a restructured healthcare system that allows them to spend time with their patients.

Regulations will be minimized to free physicians to focus on the complex processes of healing rather than running a business controlled by cut-throat industries interested only in their bottom line.

Hopefully, these issues will have been resolved and tomorrow's physicians will utilize their skills in a supportive, caring, and patient-centered environment where true healing is allowed to flourish.

* * * * *

I know and respect the work of my friend, Patricia. She is a holistic practitioner, whose work has been described in this book. She writes as follows:

Wouldn't it be wonderful if yesterday and tomorrow would combine?

An integrated mind set, encompassing body, mind, and spirit would emerge! A marriage between timeless wisdom and cutting-edge knowledge would bring about a well-rounded health care concept.

A great many medical approaches would combine: allopathic, naturopathic, homeopathic, and many others. There would be holistic health practices as well. The patient's well-being would be the primary concern of physician or practitioner. Standard care would be provided by a combined medical system of complementary and main stream medical doctors and health care professionals. There would be no more competition among those whose purpose is to 'Do no harm' and aid the patient in the healing process.

This consolidation would integrate all existing methods and modalities regarding health care into one service for the good of mankind. Everyone would benefit. Doctor and patient would be on the same team, discussing decisions and the options available for care and treatment.

Part of the routine check-up would be simply to listen intently to the patient. Most people know their own body and have some insight regarding their health concerns.

In ancient civilizations many knew how to diagnose and treat by studying the body and by using tried and true remedies to heal and cure. 'Not always' you say: even today with all the modern tools for diagnosis, mistakes are made.

There are various different modalities, many mentioned in this book, that address health and healing and several methods that involve working with the subtle energies that surround the body. Today many people continue to successfully use herbs, remedies and oils that have been used for centuries, some dating back to biblical times.

Treating the symptom instead of the cause would become history.

If a patient presented with a headache, finding the cause would be paramount, not prescribing for the headache (the symptom). In tomorrow's idealistic methods of holistic health care, 'tomorrow's physician' would always understand that the whole person must always be considered--- body, mind, and spirit.

Pain, discomfort, or disease may be caused by emotional issues as well as physical trauma. The cause or the complaint presented would be determined by methods known and understood by 'tomorrow's physician'. An integrative system encompassing all methods available would be standard procedure.

This holistic method of treating patients coupled with all the wonderful modern equipment of today's society, medical research and the knowledge of so many brilliant scholars in the medical field would be the norm for health care.

Many doctors today are using this approach. In some countries there are hospitals dedicated totally to holistic health practices, with the understanding that there are many ways to approach health and wellness.

A medical field that would not be policed by insurance and agencies that have revenue foremost in their operational goal would be non-existent. A fair practice would emerge that allowed patients to be treated as the physician sees fit for as long and as often as the treatment is needed for the good of the patient.

Health care that understands the needs of the patient and encourages medical professionals to spend quality time with their patients and staff would be encouraged.

No one would profit from pharmaceuticals except the companies that produced them, the researchers that work for those companies, and the pharmacies that sold them.

In health care, government would not be involved in decision making A combination of medical and alternative professionals would create a board to make decisions for health care workers, hospitals, and patients involved in treatment.

Doctors would practice without the fear of being sued. And the high price of insurance would be made affordable to professionals and patients alike. Insurance companies could not dictate regarding treatment or duration of hospital stay. All valid methods of healing would be recognized as part of the complete insurance package.

Many possibilities and innovative ideas and concepts combine to make these thoughts wonderfully challenging. 'Tomorrow's physician' could bring about an ideal situation for both patient and doctor.

I look forward to a future when a health care system arises from the knowledge of past centuries to combine with the present and all that is yet to come. It will be of benefit to all. 'Tomorrow's Physician' will be equipped with the tools needed to care for patients holistically with the best of ancient and modern medicine at his fingertips.

* * * * *

My friend Renate, whose reflexology treatments have helped so many, expresses the first thought of a number of those whom we asked about the physician we hope to see in the world of tomorrow:

I would want him or her to be like the doctors of yesterday, those who were familiar to us in small towns where the patients and their families were well known to the doctor. Like them, the doctor of the future would realize that the patient knows himself better than anyone else and would give him the benefit of a doubt. The doctor would listen patiently and then think before prescribing drugs.

A good example would be myself. Many years ago, I had terrible itching in my ears, which was driving me crazy. I went to an ENT clinic and the doctor gave me one medication after the other, but none of them worked. Finally he sent me to the head of the clinic, who gave me a mixture of vinegar and alcohol. Voila! It was like manna from heaven! Relief at last!

So the old-time doctor would probably have tried the simple remedy first, and then the medications if necessary. The doctor of the future will do the same if he so chooses; he won't have to protect himself from being sued. For both tomorrow's patient and physician, insurance will be a benefit, never a source of anxiety.

Tomorrow's physician will not be so quick to prescribe expensive drugs that may subject the patient to dangerous side effects. He/She will be aware of simple home remedies that are usually safe and that may nip a problem in the bud at minimal cost. He/She will have the freedom to tell patients about natural remedies that are safe and inexpensive and that have cured cancer or other serious problems.

Tomorrow's physicians will use their knowledge of other healing modalities to which patients in need of alternative or complementary help might be referred. He/she would trust other practitioners to supplement or supplant the treatment originally offered or supplied.

* * * * *

Those who are served by tomorrow's physicians will bring to them their trust and respect. They will experience shared responsibility for their health with those whom they consult. Tomorrow's physicians, along with their patients, will know and understand the basic premises of good nutrition, sufficient water, and helpful supplements. They will value the body's needs for adequate sleep and exercise. Advice and guidance in observing basic health premises will be offered when they are needed.

The patients of tomorrow will welcome the individualized advice and recommendations given them. These will be based on the initial and subsequent consultations shared by patient and physician. The patient will be accustomed to bringing complete and honest self observations and reporting the results of previous advice given and of efforts undertaken on his/her own behalf. Questions posed by the patient will be relevant and insightful. Honest answers will be expected and supplied on the basis of mutual understanding of what may be required for the patient's well-being.

Tomorrow's physician may advise help for a patient based on wonderful modern discoveries and inventions. Or referral may be made to practitioners of ancient arts that are still available, and knowledge of natural helps long known and yet utilized by modern man. And there will be new ones yet to be discovered. To these, tomorrow's physician will add the ever-valued human component of respect and concern for fellow human beings.

CHAPTER TWENTY

Health of Body, Mind and Spirit

When I set about writing a book about wellness, I had a sketchy initial plan. It grew as I delved into its various aspects. One thing led to another as I realized how much I had assimilated as my own in a long life. And how much there still remained to be encountered and explored!

I began on a very physical level with my mother's sensible dictum: "You are what you eat." Those down to earth words have lived in my kitchen and have led me beyond that to explore roads and pathways little anticipated or traveled before. My mother's practical kitchen wisdom has found renewed application with regard to the world of thoughts.

Like so many others I have been deeply absorbed in the accounts of Dr Emoto's research work with water crystals. I have been fascinated by the beautiful pictures of them he has shared with us in his books. What is revealed and intimated by these crystals has engaged the interest and wonder of learned men and women in diverse fields all over the world. To unsophisticated folk like myself they have also opened new avenues of insight about the nature of water and the effect upon it of human words and thoughts.

As a teacher, I have especially loved his work with children. When he has shown children the beautiful crystals produced by water that has been frozen after being exposed to written or spoken words, he also shows them the disagreeable forms produced by quite different words.

The children see that words like "it's going to be all right." "You tried hard." have produced beautiful crystals. Others, like "It's hopeless" or "You're stupid" produce ugly things. Then they are given the opportunity to see for themselves what their words can do. They are shown two glass jars filled with boiled rice. To the rice in the first jar they are told to say nice things. The rice in the second jar is to hear only unkind words spoken by the children.

The youngsters wait with excited interest and suspense the required number of days until it becomes quite clear when they look at the boiled rice just what has happened. The rice to which only kind words were spoken, like "You're nice", "I really like you." has become a lovely golden color, and has a pleasant smell. The rice to which ugly words were spoken is black, rotted, and smells awful.

It is not difficult to encourage the children to understand what has been dramatically demonstrated to them about the power of human thought and word. As adults we can understand still more.

As for me, it is the nature of thoughts themselves that has engrossed and captivated my attention. I remember the unforgettable experience I had as a child of nine in the course of my third grade school year. The teacher read to the class the book that has become for thousands of children "my favorite book of all." Bless the dear woman, she read us *The Secret Garden!*

In breathless silence we lived with Mary, who was unhealthy and bored with life when she came from India to live in her uncle's big house on the English moorland. Her thoughts were sour and hateful. And those, of the boy Colin, whom she discovered also living in the big house were no better. He too hated other people. He was sickly, bossy and fearful of dying. The story tells of how these two unlovely children meet. It tells of the wonderful part played by the secret garden in their lives. It tells of how this magical place touches the lives of all who find their way to it. The tale captures every heart. It was worth going to school to hear the next chapter of this special book!

Interwoven in the tale is the author's knowledge and conviction about thoughts. The third grade was introduced to Colin's father, a broken hearted, dark-tempered man who mourned the loss of his wife, Colin's mother. He had locked the door to the secret garden, buried the key and gone far away from England with his sad thoughts.

The third grade heard that thoughts are very powerful, that it had been found out that they were "just as powerful as electric batteries" and that they could be as bad for you as poison, or as good for you as sunshine. A bad thought could be as bad as a scarlet fever germ, and if you let it stay inside you, you might never be able to get it out.

It is not always easy to get rid of bad thoughts.

The third grade was relieved and happy when all the negative thoughts were conquered, and when all things worked together for good.

Now these many years later I was pleasantly surprised to find my old favorite on a DVD at the library. Would the story be spoiled by scenes and characters quite different from those that still lived in my memory? Would the unforgettable quality of the story have been preserved?

I was not disappointed. The complete text of the book is presented, in each of its 27 chapters in large clear print centered on a pretty border of green, growing things. Before each chapter there are non-specific pictures of flowers that might grow in a special garden. The text is read aloud by a gifted reader who clearly loves and understands the story. The text can be read along with her voice. Or one can choose just to listen, or just to read for that matter. I loved listening and following the words of the text. It was a peaceful and happy experience, respite from the tumult of the present-day world.

I perceived that other adults had checked out this DVD. Of course they may have children. Perhaps they want to see how the old story has been handled in a new version Do they wish to relive the delight once experienced as a child? Or is it another example of what we have seen in the "Star Wars" series---the longing for the triumph of good over evil ? Perhaps a part of all of these.

One thing is certain. The author, Frances Hodgson Burnett, was a gifted writer. The reader, or the listener, must take unconscious delight in her words. She also possessed an important wisdom. And she knew how to incorporate it quietly into her words without forcing it as something to be learned. The power of thoughts was inherent in what she had to say. Every child could grasp the importance of thoughts and their unrelenting effects.

We took that wisdom with us from the third grade. In many of us it became a living part of our being. It was unspoken, but very real, unlike the lessons in morality to which we might have been exposed elsewhere.

* * * * *

Some of the lessons in morality came from the church. My parents did not talk about religion, but they went to church sometimes, and seemed to think it appropriate for us to attend Sunday School. We started to go when a friend of the family provided transportation, Some of the things I heard there didn't make sense to me. I thought I would be given the answers to my questions when I became fourteen and was enrolled in a confirmation class. "Now I will know," thought I.

The confirmation class was given a great deal of dogmatic information; some of it we had to learn by heart. The pastor explained it all so that we would understand it. "That's what he says it means," thought I. "But if that's what it means, I don't believe it." I kept these feelings to myself, and was duly confirmed without having to divulge my heresy.

In the ensuing years there were youth groups, conducted by handsome young men who were assistant pastors. They tried earnestly to meet our needs, but I felt no more satisfied by their answers to my questions than I had felt before.

Some of the hymns we sang were filled with strange assertions. I sang along with them nonetheless. The best of them, which appeared with reassuring regularity was called the Doxology and was sung in praise of God. It is the kind of song you sing when you are surrounded by fresh air, sunshine, cooling winds, and fragrant growing things. The children sang it joyfully in *The Secret Garden* once they all had good thoughts:

> "Praise God from Whom all blessings flow.
> Praise Him all creatures here below.
> Praise Him above ye heavenly host.
> Praise Father, Son and Holy Ghost."

I was reassured some years later when I read the words of an Anglican priest spoken to someone like myself with unanswered questions: "My dear, of course you must believe in God, in spite of what the clergy tell you."

I never doubted the existence of God, though I could not impute to the Creator the arbitrary actions in which so many seemed to believe. My parents themselves provided the best examples of how a human being should be expected to behave. My mother's unfailing love gave us all support in every worthy endeavor. My father's support of those who were in need. outside the family was something we only knew about years after it occurred. Also a well-kept secret were the hours he spent reading the Bible to his illiterate buddies in the trenches of France during the First World War.

* * * * *

As a young adult I returned full of joy and thanksgiving to visit my relatives in Denmark. The difficult war years were behind them, and I could again be with the beloved cousin who had always meant so much to me as a child. I would not have dreamed that it would be she who could answer the questions I had bottled up within me for so many years.

Once having grasped this to be the case, there was no end to the questions that poured from my lips. We talked in a Danish ditch among the bluebells and other wild flowers. We talked in the kitchen as we washed and dried the dishes. We talked over the breakfast in bed supplied by a loving aunt.

Later we talked in my cousin's little house near Copenhagen. It was the place in which she had sheltered Sister Rosa, the refugee from Hitler's Third Reich. From Sister Rosa my cousin had heard the words: "Do not forget that nothing that happens to us is accidental."

Now I learned that the answers to my questions, so readily supplied by my cousin, had come from the book *In the Light of Truth, the Grail Message*. A few months later I held that book in my own hands. It became my most precious possession. To paraphrase the words of a young friend with whom I discussed it years later, "It's the one thing I'd grab before rushing out if my house was on fire." I had longed for something more than organized religion had provided. Now it was mine.

* * * * *

My new book disclosed a totally new world to me. Its many chapters held my complete attention. Ideas that I had taken for granted were presented in an entirely different way. Concepts I had never examined seriously became significant parts of a meaningful whole. The world as I had previously known it was seen in a new light. I could not read this book in the same carefree manner in which I had swallowed so many books all through my life. Nor was it like any college text I had ever studied. It seemed to give and give to me and yet to make far-reaching demands.

I wanted to speak with my cousin about all this. Yet in another way I did not wish to speak with anyone about it. It was mine alone, and every hour I gave to its reading made it more fully mine.

The information about thoughts impressed me deeply. I fancied myself to be familiar with thoughts. I remembered what I learned in the third grade. I had spent four years in college. Thoughts had preceded the writing of texts and examinations. I had been admonished to think clearly. I had learned how to teach children to do likewise. Thoughts always initiated some specific physical action or produced some visible, tangible result. Once that was accomplished you could forget about the thinking part.

Now I read and understood that thoughts are as real as rocks, flowers, trees, or bicycles and cars, for that matter. They are as real and tangible as any other physical thing. They have forms that some people can see. And thoughts that are alike are attracted to each other. I imagined good thoughts clustering like great castles of cumulus clouds and evil thoughts coming together in threatening heaps of black clouds filled with lightning and thunder.

Thoughts, I realized, are like that, but they are much more powerful.

Even the loveliest cloud castles are soon forgotten. And the most violent thunderstorm is dissipated. Thoughts endure, to bring blessing or disaster. With our thoughts we contribute to the kind of world in which we live.

Now when I contemplate Dr. Emoto's rice experiment with the children I am overwhelmed by the power of thoughts. Like the water-soaked rice in the glass jar, I too can absorb thoughts that have access from the world around me. (My body is over 60% water!) Some of it is beyond my control. Our atmosphere is filled with thoughts carried on radio waves, the waves of e-mail, the websites on the internet, cell phones and other modern means of communication.

Other thoughts or sounds can be controlled by my volition. Like the food I eat, the thoughts I choose to keep can become part of me.

I am what I choose to consume. The modern world is heaped like a banquet table with assorted offerings for my consumption. My eyes can be riveted all day, if I choose, on the empty images transmitted by television. I can seek out similar emptiness in modern art. My ears can be filled with the raucous sounds of meaningless music. I can read books that keep me in suspense with tales or romance, crime, violence, and lust. I can choose habits that ultimately make me a slave to them.

I can find much to give me personal, physical pleasure. There are many things that do not weary the mind, or call upon the effort involved when the inner self is required to respond.

There are other choices that one might term "a lot of trouble." I am free to make those choices too. I can nourish the inner self with what are called "good thoughts." The specific outcome of those thoughts will depend on the individual circumstances in which each of us lives. What is easy for you may be a lot of trouble for me. And vice versa! Each of us must learn to choose thoughts that make us strong, confident and grateful for life and living, regardless of the cost. Or we can opt for thoughts that make us hopeless, depressed, and lethargic.

The thoughts we choose can be destructive, or they can contribute to physical wellness and the wellness of the inner self that we call soul, or the spirit.

I am aware of the multiple hazards to which we are exposed on our planet. I know that many can in the blink of an eye be made to feel like helpless victims. I know that we cannot expect the Creator to intervene to prevent or ameliorate our woes. Yet I know that we have been given the power of thought to access in prayer the great thought centers of strength and comfort, or to pray for intervention on behalf of others.

Our thoughts of genuine love and gratitude for even the smallest things are of no small account. They are significant. They constitute an essential part of our wellness. Whatever we can do to improve the quality of our physical health is important. It makes us feel good. In like manner good thoughts, whether given or received, also make us feel good. To feel good contributes to our becoming able to <u>be</u> good. And that goal is something that all of us can hope to achieve!

* * * * *

Good thoughts may accompany cheerful kitchen experiences, the preparation of health-giving food. They may relate to discovering natural supplements to restore or maintain our health.

They may be associated with the joy of movement. Surely they are present in the effort of eliminating a bad habit that can interfere with good health and in the satisfaction of overcoming it.

There are good thoughts in experiencing the services of health practitioners who know and respect the body. We exchange good thoughts with physicians who know and understand our physical needs. Good thoughts support our emotional needs and help us to deal with them. The wisdom we find in meaningful books engenders and nourishes our progress as human beings.

We can learn to stretch and exercise body and mind. We can learn to use wisely the riches of the planet on which we live. We can learn how to give and receive love, and how to express gratitude. It is not always easy. Experience in a long earth-life has taught me that nonetheless we can learn to be well in body, mind and spirit. It is a responsibility that each of us, in his or her own way, can learn to accept.

There is so much available to teach us the art of wellness. With all its perils, its hazards, its chaos, this earth still has many treasures. They are alive and intact waiting for us to find them. They invite us to grow, to live and to be.

BIBLIOGRAPHY

This list is designed to be of help to those looking for their own adventures in wellness. Included are titles of books that have been personally useful to me in gaining or maintaining health.

Librarians can be very helpful in directing you to books that may be right for you. My own local library has been quick to order titles not available on our own shelves, from inter-library loan.

Those who are book-buyers will want to get acquainted with **Better World Books.** This wonderful organization has a vast assortment of new and used books. Whatever you choose is sent quickly and without shipping charges. Furthermore, for every one you order a book is sent to some place in the world where books are desperately needed! **Better World Books** is easily accessed on the internet.

"You Are What You Eat!"

Cook Right For Your Type
   By Dr. Peter J. D'Adamo
   C.P. Putnam's Sons 1998
   Includes more than 200 Original Recipes as well as individualized 30-Day meal plans for Staying Healthy, Living Longer, and Achieving Your Ideal Weight.

The Acid-Alkaline Diet for Optimum Health
   By Chrisopher Vasey
   Healing Arts Press, Rochester, Vermont 1999
   "Restore your Health by Creating Balance in Your Diet"

The Get With the Program! Guide to Good Eating
By Bob Greene
"An effective and enjoyable approach to good health, good eating, and weight loss that you can trust."

"Go Out and Play"

Five Tibetans
By Christopher S. Kilham
Healing Arts Press 1994
"Five Dynamic Exercises for Health, Energy and Personal Power"

The Five Rites of Rejuvenation
By Peter Kelder
Now called **The Eye of Revelation**
This is the original book that sparked worldwide; interest in "The Five Tibetans"

Lillias! Yoga Gets Better with Age
By Lillias Folan
Rodale Books, July 2005
Popular on TV, Lillias introduced yoga to millions
200 illustrations. Postures adapted to be safe for any age.
Down to earth, likable.

Health Advice from the Twelfth Century

Hildegard of Bingen's Medicine
By Dr. Wighard
Strehloh & Gottfried Herzka, M.D.
Folk Wisdom Series Bear & Company
Santa Fe, New Mexico 1988

The First Modern Physician

Paracelsus, His Mystical and Medical Philosophy
By Manly P. Hall
The Philosophical Research Society, Inc. 1964

Health Through God's Pharmacy
By Maria Treben
Publisher: Ennsthaler Steyr 2009
Translated from the German.
Advice and Proven Cures with Medicinal Herbs

A Revolutionary Discovery

Transfer Factors
By Rita Elkins. M.H.
Woodland Publishing, Pleasant Grove, Utah
"Nature's State-of-the-Art Immune Fortifiers

Ancient Health Help in New Hands

Essential Oils Desk Reference
Compiled by Essential Science Publishing
"To all those who seek truth, light and wisdom. After all it is their hearts that turn to the information in this book."

Quick Reference Guide for Using Essential Oils
Compiled by Connie and Alan Higley
Abundant Health, Spanish Fork, UT 84660

Healing at Our Fingertips

Body Reflexology
By Mildred Carter and Tammy Weber
Reward Books, A member of Penguin Group (USA)
"Healing at Your Fingertips"

Hand Reflexology: Key to Perfect Health
By Mildred Carter
Parker Publishing Company, West Nyack, NY
"Revealing in this book – amazing health secret said to trigger dynamic healing power of body's mysterious 'nerve circuits'"

The Touch of Healing

The Touch of Healing
By Alice Burmeister with Tom Monte
Bantam Books New York Toronto London Sydney Auckland
"Energizing Body, Mind and Spirit with the Art of Jin Shin Jtutzu"

The Healing Codes

The Healing Code
By Alex Loyd, PhD, ND and Ben Johnson, MD, DO, NMD
Intermedia Publishing Group, Inc.
"Discover the revolutionary formula that heals the source of illness and disease, even success and relationship issues."

The Miracle of Water

Your Body's Many Cries for Water
By F. Batmanghelidj, M.D.
Global Health Solutions, Inc.
P.O. Box 3189 Falls Church, VA 20043 YSA
"You Are Not Sick, You Are Thirsty! Don't treat thirst with medications"
"A Preventive and Self=Education Manual"

Health Hazards in the World Around Us

Outsmart Your Cancer
By Tanya Harter Pierce, M.A., MFCC
Thoughtworks Publishing
Stateline, Nevada, 2009
"Alternative Non-Toxic Treatments That Work"

How To Survive (and Thrive) In A Toxic World
By Jeannette Russell
"A User's Guide to Avoiding Chemicals for Radiant Health and a Clean Home Environment"

90 Years Young!

Health of Body, Mind and Spirit

The Grail Message, In the Light of Truth
  By Abd-ru-shin (Oskar Ernst Bernhardt, 1875-1941)
  Grail Foundation Press 800-427-9217
  Download at minimal cost from
  www.grailfoundationpress.com